# HEMP OIL

Ease pain and promote healing with CBD oil. Learn where to buy it, how to use it, and the conditions it treats.

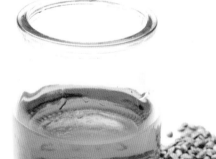

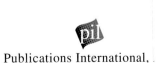

Publications International,

D1307929

**Written by:** Sheryl DeVore

**Additional material:** Lisa Brooks

**Photography:** Shutterstock.com and Wikimedia Commons

ISBN: 978-1-64030-731-5

Manufactured in China.

8 7 6 5 4 3 2 1

# Table of Contents

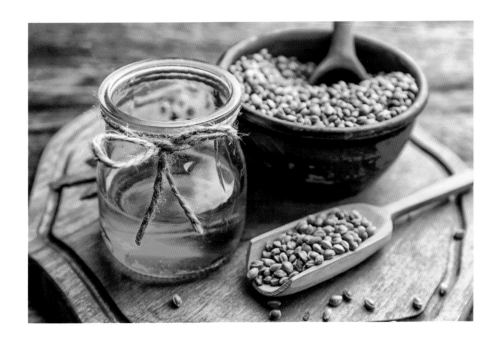

# Introduction

Maybe you have a chronic health condition, and your son or daughter—or even your doctor—has recommended that you consider a prescription for medical marijuana. Maybe you went to lunch at a friend's house, and she blithely sprinkled hemp seeds on her salad, and you wondered if you were going to get a high. Maybe your sister says that she's started taking CBD oil to treat her arthritis, and you wonder what that is. However you found your way to this book, our goal is to provide you with answers to the often confusing world of hemp, medical marijuana, hemp oil and seeds, CBD oil, THC, CBD, cannabinoids, and more.

In chapter 1, The Basics of Hemp and Marijuana, learn about the history of hemp and marijuana in the world and the United States. Learn about the different strains of the cannabis plant and the many uses of hemp, as well as how and when it became illegal—a relatively recent historic development.

In chapter 2, The Endocannabinoid System, delve into this important body system that helps regulate homeostasis. Substances in the cannabis plant such as THC (the substance in marijuana that causes a high) and CBD (cannabidiol, which does not cause a high) interact with this system, affecting your mood and health.

In chapter 3, Medical Marijuana Today, take a look at the current legal status of cannabis use at the federal and state levels.

In chapter 4, Hemp Seeds, find out about these nutritious little gems and how you can incorporate them in your diet.

In Chapter 5, CBD: A Primer, learn the ins and outs of CBD oil made from hemp, from how it's made to its many forms such tinctures, salves, and edibles. Learn about the questions you should ask before taking CBD oil, from dosage to side effects to drug interactions.

In the final section, Medical Conditions, we explore how CBD oil has been used—or might be used—for specific medical conditions that vary from ADHD to arthritis to heart disease to anxiety. Examine the scientific evidence—or, in some cases, the questions that remain—as you consider whether you should consider taking CBD oil to treat your health condition.

*Hemp Oil* offers a comprehensive view of the cannabis plant and its potential uses, focusing particularly on the many uses of CBD oil. Find out how it might help you.

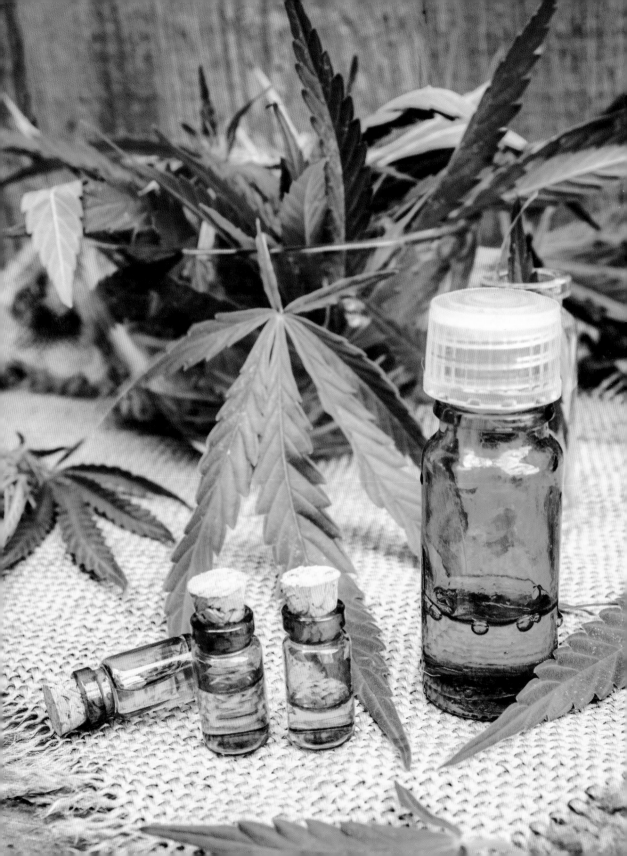

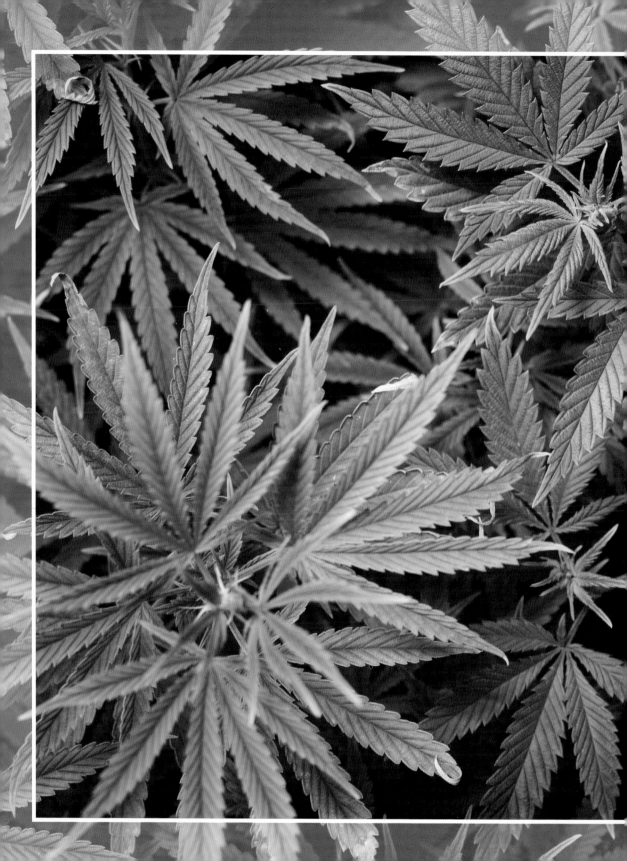

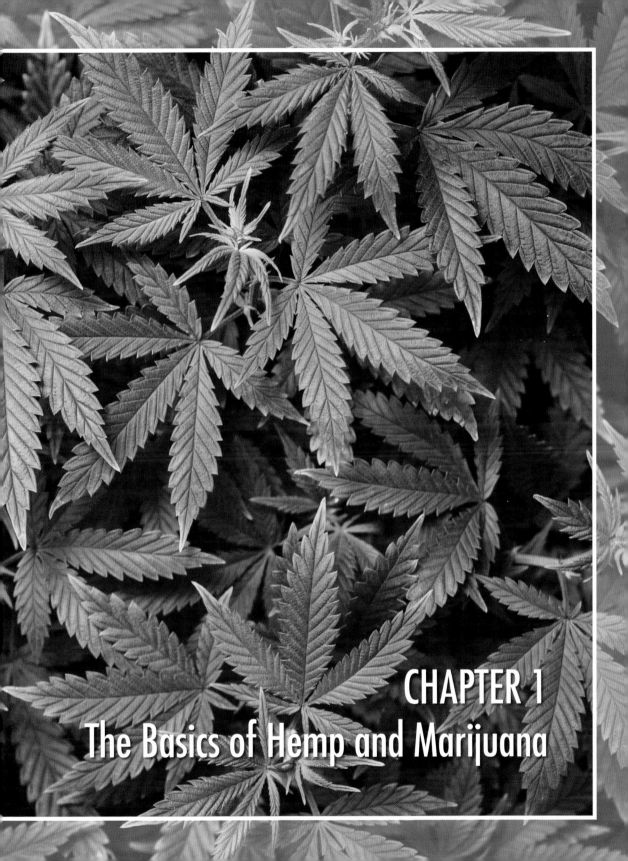

# CHAPTER 1
# The Basics of Hemp and Marijuana

# The History of Hemp

Medical marijuana has been in the news in the past decade, as have—in a quieter way—hemp and CBD oil. So let's start with the basics. There's more than one type of cannabis plant, and the uses of the different types go far beyond medicine or pain relief. *Cannabis sativa* is the plant that is known for its medicinal and psychoactive properties; but a subspecies, *Cannabis sativa L.*—the "L" in honor of botanist Carl Linnaeus—is more commonly known as hemp. This species of cannabis has little to none of the psychoactive properties of *Cannabis sativa*, making it much more useful for manufacturing products such as cloth and oil.

## What Hemp Can Do

As our forebears discovered, this amazing plant has a myriad of uses: Hemp seeds are edible and can be used in breads, cereals, or as protein powder. They can even be used to create a vegan "milk." The oil of the seed is useful for ink, paint, cosmetics, and personal care products like lotions and soap. Hemp stalks produce the fibers that have been used for thousands of years to create clothing, paper, shoes, carpets, and rope. More recently, hemp has even been used to create building materials, such as insulating blocks and plaster used in houses, and composite panels used in automobiles.

It would seem that hemp can do just about everything, but there's one thing it can't do: hemp can't give you the "high" associated with *Cannabis sativa*, due to its low concentration of the psychoactive substance tetrahydrocannabinol, or THC. Regardless, the 1937 Marijuana Tax Act began restricting the growth and sale of all forms of cannabis, and in 1970, the Controlled Substances Act categorized both *Cannabis sativa* and *Cannabis sativa L.* as "Schedule I" drugs—despite the fact that hemp lacks any psychoactive properties!

For decades, growing any type of cannabis in the U.S. was illegal—even perfectly innocuous hemp—so most of the hemp used in the country was imported. Because of its prohibition, many people have been unaware of the amazing uses this plant provides and have often equated hemp with its medicinal cousin.

But over the last decade, regulations have slowly started to change, and it is now legal to grow hemp in more than a dozen states. Not only that, but more than half of U.S. states have now legalized marijuana for medical use; perhaps hemp is not the only cannabis plant that has been unfairly maligned. On the coming pages, we'll delve into the history of hemp and marijuana.

One-hundred milliliters of hemp biodiesel made from hemp seeds, hemp stalks, and alcohol.

A botanical illustration of the *Cannabis sativa L.* plant. A) Flowering Male Plant, B) Seed-Bearing Female Plant, 1) Male Flower, 2) Pollen Sac, 3) Pollen Sac (different angle), 4) Pollen Grain of Sac, 5) Female Flower With Cover Petal, 6) Female Flower Without Cover Petal, 7) Female Fruit (cross section), 8) Fruit With Cover Petal, 9) Fruit Without Cover Petal, 10) Fruit Without Cover Petal (different angle), 11) Fruit Without Cover Petal (cross section), 12) Fruit Without Cover Petal (longitudinal cross section), 13) Seed Without Hull

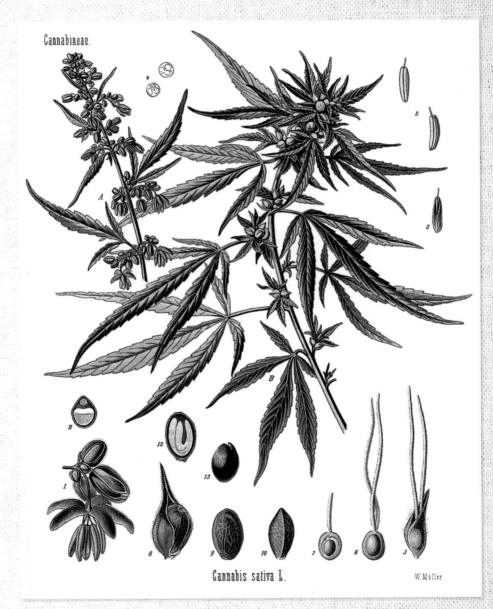

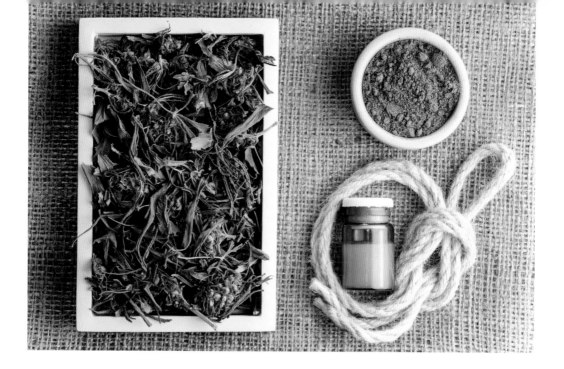

# Hemp and Marijuana in History

Hemp's history goes back thousands of years. In fact, the Cannabis plant is actually one of the world's oldest cultivated crops, with its origin going all the way back to the development of agriculture itself. Hemp was one of the first plants to be spun into a fiber, and these fibers have been discovered in pottery at archeological sites dating back 10,000 years in what is now Taiwan. Around 6000 BC, the Chinese began using hemp seeds and oil for food, and over the next two thousand years, they learned to weave the fiber into fine textiles. Rope made of hemp was commonly used throughout China, Russia, and Greece by 200 BC. But the Chinese, not content to stop with rope and cloth, next invented hemp paper; eventually, the Arabs learned this technique, as well.

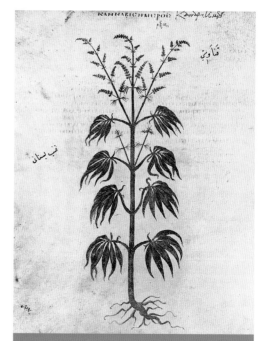

A botanical illustration of *Cannabis sativa* from a Byzantine Greek illuminated manuscript of Dioscorides' *De Materia Medica*. This manuscript was made in 515 AD in Constantinople for the daughter of one of the last Western Roman Emperors, Anicius Olybrius.

Archeologists believe marijuana's use goes back at least 12,000 years. Cannabis probably originated in the area that is now Mongolia, but seeds dating back to 3000 BC have also been found in Siberia and parts of China, and mummified marijuana has been found in the ancient tombs of Chinese nobles.

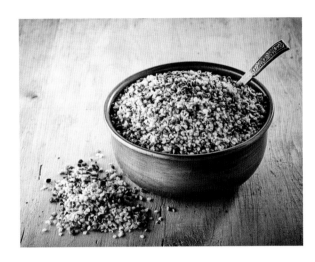

The oldest record of marijuana's medicinal use dates back to 4000 BC, when the plant was used for its anesthetic properties. By 1000 BC, cannabis had made its way to the Middle East and India, where it was prized for its ability to relieve anxiety. It was even mentioned in an ancient sacred Hindu text called *Atharvaveda*—which translates to "Science of Charms"—where it was dubbed "sacred grass."

From South Asia, marijuana's popularity spread to the Greeks and Romans, and its value as a medicinal plant really began to take hold. Roman naturalist Pliny the Elder wrote of its analgesic effects in his book *Naturalis Historia* ("Natural History"); Roman army medic Dioscorides described medical marijuana in his pharmacopoeia, *De Materia Medica* ("On Medical Material"); and famous ancient Greek physician Galen often prescribed marijuana to his patients.

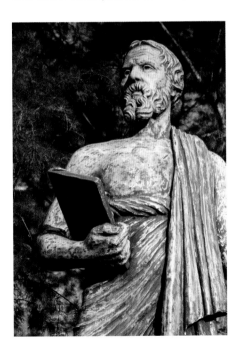

Herodotus, the Greek historian who is often considered "The Father of History," gives us one of the earliest records of marijuana use in his 440 BC manuscript, *Histories*. After an encounter with the Scythian people of Eurasia, he recounted their practice of taking baths in cannabis steam. He writes, "The Scythians, as I said, take some of this hemp-seed [presumably flowers], and, creeping under the felt coverings, throw it upon the red-hot stones; immediately it smokes, and gives out such a vapour as no Grecian vapour-bath can exceed; the Scyths, delighted, shout for joy."

Arab traders took the plant south to the Mozambique coast of Africa, and nomadic Indo-European tribes carried the plant further west, where Vikings and Germanic peoples used it as a pain reliever for childbirth and toothaches.

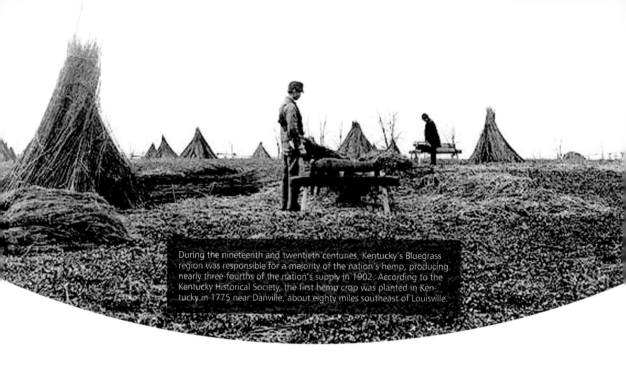

During the nineteenth and twentieth centuries, Kentucky's Bluegrass region was responsible for a majority of the nation's hemp, producing nearly three-fourths of the nation's supply in 1902. According to the Kentucky Historical Society, the first hemp crop was planted in Kentucky in 1775 near Danville, about eighty miles southeast of Louisville.

# Journey to the Americas

The journey of hemp's usefulness followed the path of medicinal marijuana, with hemp rope soon showing up in England and other parts of Europe. Hemp cloth became popular, as well, and not just with the common populace: the Merovingian queen Arnegunde was buried with her finest jewelry, and wrapped in a hemp shroud. Over the next several hundred years, hemp rope became standard on European ships—including those used by Christopher Columbus—and the fiber was in high demand. In fact, it was so prized that in 1533 King Henry VIII began fining farmers who refused to grow hemp for industrial use! Spaniards introduced hemp to South America in the mid-sixteenth century, and by the seventeenth century, the Puritans were cultivating the crop in New England.

Over the next several hundred years, marijuana enjoyed increasing popularity within the Americas. Even the first president of the United States, George Washington, grew hemp and encouraged its cultivation in the new country due to its industrial purposes. By the 1700s, medical marijuana was used in New England, and by the 1800s, the plant was commonly grown on plantations in many southern states, as well as New York and California. The plant became vitally important during World War II, when hemp was used to make uniforms, canvas, and rope. (By the way, if the word canvas has a familiar ring to it, that's because it was derived from the word cannabis— the material first used to construct it!)

Medical marijuana was even easily available for purchase throughout the United States at pharmacies and general stores. After millennia of medical use, it seemed that this versatile drug was poised to become a staple within the medical community. But as anyone can see from the decades-long debate over medical marijuana, things have not been that simple for the cannabis plant.

# Cannabis Loses Ground

As the anti-drug campaigns of the late twentieth century demonstrated, the drug fell out of favor and was considered illegal for decades; today, however, marijuana is rebounding.

But why was this time-tested, widely used plant ever criminalized to begin with? The answer dates back to 1910, when the Mexican Revolution caused great unrest in the country. Mexican immigrants began fleeing to states like Texas and Louisiana to escape the violence, and the newcomers, of course, brought their customs and culture with them. One of the customs they enjoyed was the use of marijuana as a recreational drug. Americans were used to the substance as medicine; cannabis was widely available in pharmacies across the country. But this new, recreational use of marijuana was a novel idea. In fact, even the word *marijuana* was foreign to Americans, as the word *cannabis* was always used for the popular tinctures and medicines in pharmacies.

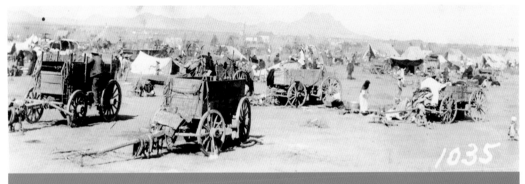

A photo, circa 1914, of refugees fleeing the violence of the Mexican Revolution.

The Spanish-speaking immigrants who arrived in the country were often met with prejudice and suspicion. And these attitudes were also expressed towards their custom of marijuana use. The media caught on to the public's distrust of Mexican immigrants, and began to rail against the foreigners, painting a picture of violent and disruptive immigrants and raising fears in Americans. Authorities began to blame the "violence" of these immigrants on their use of marijuana, calling it a "killer weed" that gave its users "superhuman strength," and warning the public that Mexicans were handing out the drug to innocent schoolchildren. Americans, unaware that this "marijuana" was the very same cannabis that sat in their medicine cabinets, were convinced that the immigrants had introduced a dangerous new drug to the country.

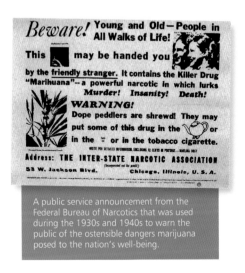

A public service announcement from the Federal Bureau of Narcotics that was used during the 1930s and 1940s to warn the public of the ostensible dangers marijuana posed to the nation's well-being.

# National Paranoia

By 1931, twenty-nine states had outlawed marijuana, even though there was no evidence that the drug was particularly dangerous. But the public's perception of the drug—fueled by fear and prejudice against the Mexican immigrants—along with propaganda like the 1936 film *Reefer Madness*, eventually led to the Marijuana Tax Act of 1937, which enacted country-wide penalties for anyone who bought or sold cannabis. And in the 1950s, federal laws were created that made the penalties even stricter: A first offense conviction for possession of marijuana could carry a sentence of two to ten years in prison and a $20,000 fine!

After thousands of years of use around the world, suddenly cannabis was reduced from hero to villain in mere decades. And just as quickly, marijuana developed a reputation—and certainly not a good one. More and more people were using the drug for recreational purposes as opposed to medicinally, and many Americans felt that "getting high" wasn't a good enough reason to con-sume cannabis. Instead of being seen as a medicinal marvel with a relatively safe track record, the drug was now considered a dangerous substance only used by drug addicts. This was despite the fact that the medicines Americans had been using for decades and the "new" drug marijuana were one and the same!

*Reefer Madness* is a propaganda film that follows the downfall of a group of high-school students who become addicted to marijuana. Many decades later, the film was rediscovered and became a cult classic as an unintentional satire.

Perhaps the worst consequence of the stereotypes and stigmas surrounding cannabis is that they have prevented many from seeing the drug as a viable medicinal remedy. Even with thousands of years of use and evidence to back up the claim of marijuana's medici-nal prowess, efforts to legalize the plant have been slow going. Some scoff at the idea that the drug is good for anything other than a "high," while others are interested in trying the remedy, but worry about the social stigma that might follow. And that's too bad, because cannabis has shown plenty of promising results when used for a host of ailments.

In recent decades, however, decriminalization and legalization have been on the upswing, and people have been rediscovering both the benefits of marijuana but also the other uses of the plant.

# Different Strains of Cannabis

If you're new to the cannabis scene, you may assume that all strains the same. But "marijuana" encompasses an entire world of different strains, which all come with their own pros and cons and affect users in different ways. Think of it like this: Chihuahuas, Huskies, and Rottweilers are all very different, but they have one thing in common: They're all dogs. But if you're looking for a dog that can comfortably nap on your lap while you watch TV, you probably won't choose a heavy Rottweiler; and if you need a good police dog, you probably won't go with a tiny Chihuahua!

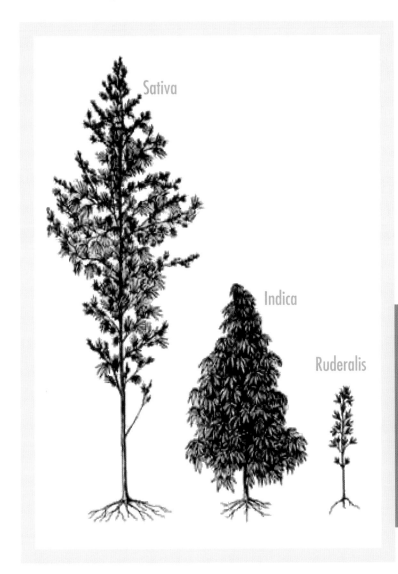

Sativa

Indica

Ruderalis

Experts say that there are at least 779 strains of marijuana in the world, but that number continually changes because cannabis growers love to experiment with crossing different plants to create new hybrids. But all of the hundreds of varieties of marijuana in the world begin with three different species: *Cannabis indica*, *Cannabis sativa*, and *Cannabis ruderalis*.

Cannabis was first identified as a monotypic species by eighteenth century botanist Carl Linnaeus. He classified the plant as *Cannabis sativa* L., but in 1785, the botanist Jean-Baptiste de Lamarck identified a second species of cannabis, which he named *Cannabis indica*. One of the major differences between the species that Lamarck noticed was that the sativa species was better for producing strong fibers, while the indica species was better for inebriation.

# Cannabis indica

Indica has traditionally been grown in parts of southeast Asia to produce *charas*, which is a type of hashish—the drug created from cannabis resin. The plant is short in stature, with broad leaves and a short flowering cycle, which makes it more ideal to colder climates with shorter growing seasons, or for indoor cultivation. Medicines produced with indica are said to induce mental and muscle relaxation, decrease nausea and pain, and increase appetite. The effects of indica are thought to be more sedating than other cannabis species, so many users consume the drug before bedtime or to relax at home.

The leaves of *Cannabis indica* are much smaller than those found on plants of the sativa species. The leaflets are very wide without much separation between them. Usually there are about seven to nine leaflets on each leaf. The color of indica's leaves remains somewhat consistent with an olive green hue. Lighter shades of green are very rare and are usually a sign of a deficiency.

# Cannabis sativa

Sativa was first cultivated near the equator, in Thailand, Mexico, and Africa. The plant is tall, with narrow leaves and a long flowering cycle, and is often grown outdoors in warmer areas with longer growing seasons. Instead of producing a sedative effect, this species is said to energize users. It can reduce anxiety and depression, increase focus and creativity, and dull chronic pain. Because of its reputation for increasing energy, users often consume sativa in social situations or during creative pursuits.

*Cannabis sativa*'s leaves are larger than those of the *Cannabis indica* or *ruderalis* species. The separations between the leaflets can be very pronounced, and there can be up to thirteen leaflets on each leaf. The color of the leaves can range from bright or lime green to an almost blackish green.

# Cannabis ruderalis

Ruderalis has traditionally been used in Russian and Mongolian folk medicine, and is thought to be especially useful for treating depression. On its own, this species is not psychoactive: ruderalis is naturally high in the compound CBD and low in the compound THC, so it's rarely grown for recreational use but prized for its medicinal properties. Ruderalis is a hardier plant than either indica or sativa, so it is able to resist disease and insects. It's also known for its very short growing season, and is mature in a matter of weeks. Because of these properties, ruderalis is often bred with indica or sativa to produce stronger, faster-growing plants with customized amounts of THC and CBD.

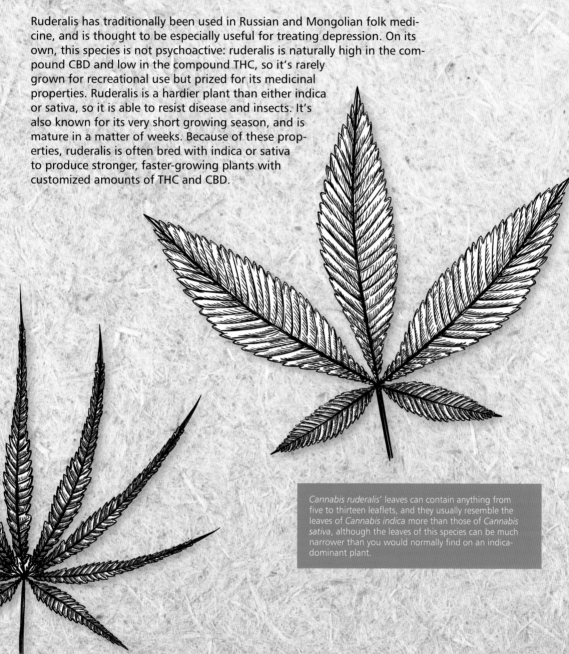

*Cannabis ruderalis*' leaves can contain anything from five to thirteen leaflets, and they usually resemble the leaves of *Cannabis indica* more than those of *Cannabis sativa*, although the leaves of this species can be much narrower than you would normally find on an indica-dominant plant.

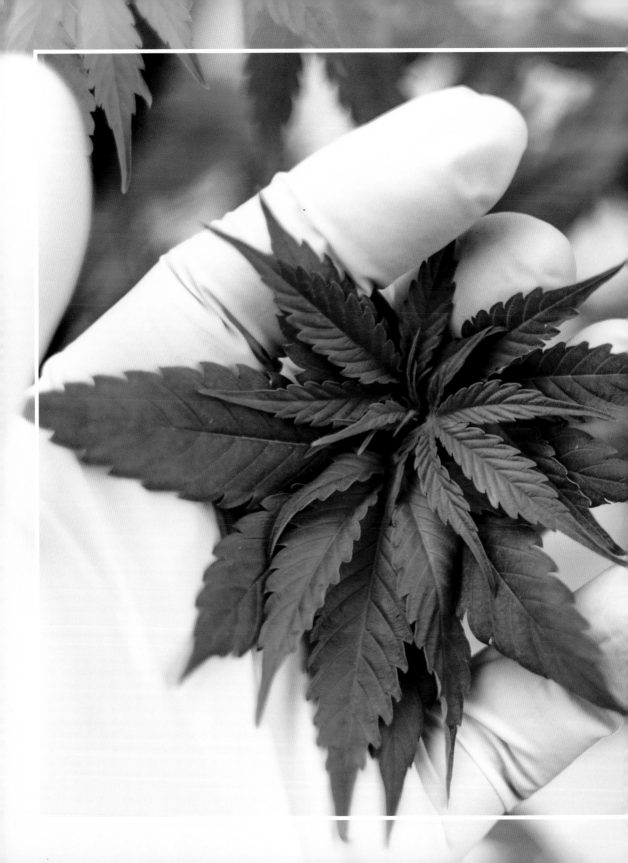

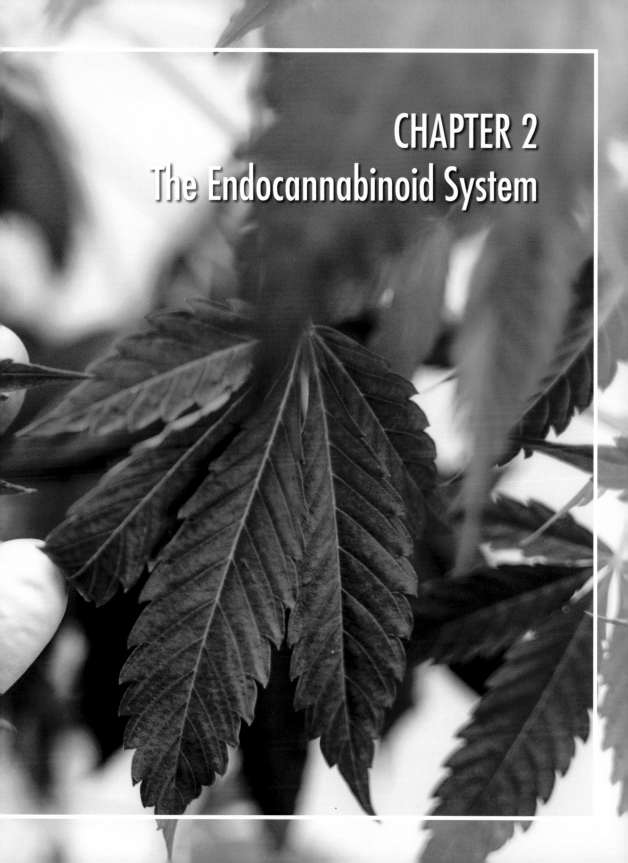

# CHAPTER 2
# The Endocannabinoid System

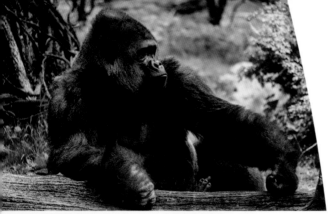

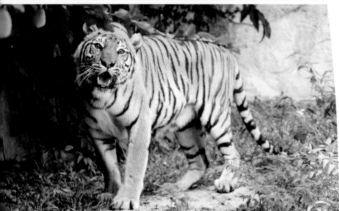

# What Is the Endocannabinoid System?

When scientists were studying how marijuana affects the body, they made a remarkable discovery in the 1990s—the endocannabinoid system or ECS.

Endocannabinoid is a big word—and the system is complex. But the ECS, named after the cannabis plant that led to its discovery, "is perhaps the most important physiologic system involved in establishing and maintaining human health," wrote Dr. Dustin Sulak in a recent online article. Dr. Sulak is an integrative medicine physician in Maine with a doctorate in osteopathic medicine and the founder of healer.com

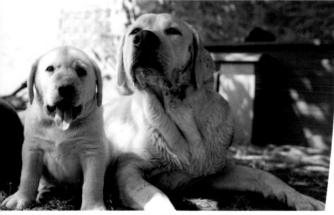

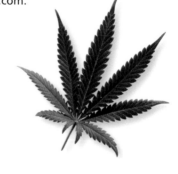

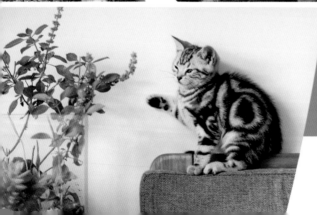

Humans aren't the only ones with the ECS. Animals with backbones such as gorillas, tigers, and your pet dog or cat have the ECS as well. Even tiny sea creatures have been shown to possess this system, and biologists believe animals that lived more than 600 million years ago had the ECS.

# What the ECS Does

This system is crucial in maintaining and regulating what biologists call homeostasis. The ECS helps our bodies maintain proper temperature and blood pressure, the correct balance of fluids, a good-working memory and mood, the ability to sleep, and more. When something goes awry, either within the body or externally, the ECS kicks in to return the body to homeostasis.

The system includes natural occurring substances called cannabinoids, which are also present in plants such as *Cannabis sativa*, from which marijuana is made. The cannabinoids in the human body are called endocannabinoids and those in plants are called phytocannabinoids.

Within our bodies are receptors that react with the cannabinoids to do their work to maintain homeostasis. When changes occur, these receptors get activated to do their jobs.

Countless cannabinoid receptors are located throughout the body, including in the nervous system and in various organs. In the brain alone, for example, they're found in the amygdala, which regulates emotions; the cerebellum, which regulates motor functioning; and the hippocampus, which regulates the ability to learn; among many others.

The receptors are located on the surface of cells. One of the main receptors is called CB1, which works in the brain and central nervous system. The other main receptor, called CB2, works with the peripheral nervous system and controls your body's immune system. It's also recently been found to work in the brain. Scientists are researching other types of cannabinoid receptors within the body.

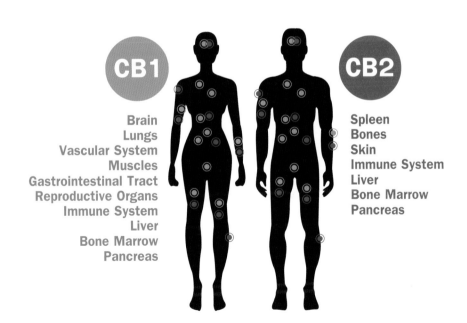

**CB1**

Brain
Lungs
Vascular System
Muscles
Gastrointestinal Tract
Reproductive Organs
Immune System
Liver
Bone Marrow
Pancreas

**CB2**

Spleen
Bones
Skin
Immune System
Liver
Bone Marrow
Pancreas

# THC, CBD, and More Cannabinoids

Scientists first discovered the chemical THC, or tetrahydrocannabinol, contained in marijuana in the 1960s. That led to research on what type of receptors are in the body that interact with THC, and then the discovery of the ECS.

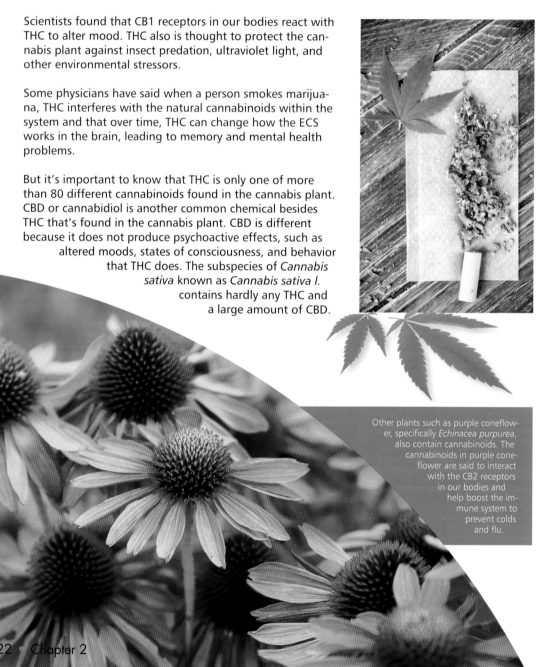

Scientists found that CB1 receptors in our bodies react with THC to alter mood. THC also is thought to protect the cannabis plant against insect predation, ultraviolet light, and other environmental stressors.

Some physicians have said when a person smokes marijuana, THC interferes with the natural cannabinoids within the system and that over time, THC can change how the ECS works in the brain, leading to memory and mental health problems.

But it's important to know that THC is only one of more than 80 different cannabinoids found in the cannabis plant. CBD or cannabidiol is another common chemical besides THC that's found in the cannabis plant. CBD is different because it does not produce psychoactive effects, such as altered moods, states of consciousness, and behavior that THC does. The subspecies of *Cannabis sativa* known as *Cannabis sativa I.* contains hardly any THC and a large amount of CBD.

Other plants such as purple coneflower, specifically *Echinacea purpurea*, also contain cannabinoids. The cannabinoids in purple coneflower are said to interact with the CB2 receptors in our bodies and help boost the immune system to prevent colds and flu.

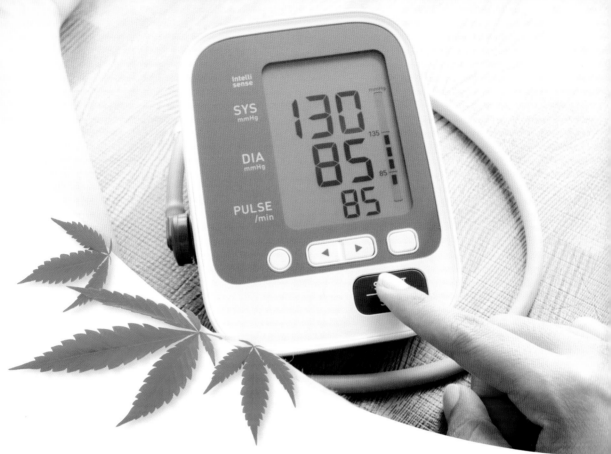

# The ECS and Your Health

There's much more to learn about these substances found in plants and in the human body and how they work with the ECS. Biologists are just on the threshold of learning how medicines might be developed based on that knowledge.

For example, they are studying how certain disorders such as diabetes, high blood pressure, liver disease, migraine, and irritable bowel syndrome could be a result of a disrupted ECS.

What they know for certain is that ECS in humans contains three important components: the naturally occurring endocannabinoids, the receptors that work with them, and the enzymes that break down the cannabinoids when they are no longer needed. Much more needs to be learned about how these enzymes work with cannabinoids inside the body as well as those that come from plants.

Scientists, biologists, and physicians know that understanding the complex ECS will take more time and research. After all, it was only discovered a few decades ago. Still, it points to new considerations in treating humans with various ailments. Based on the latest information and clinical studies, some physicians believe that proper dosages of cannabis in certain forms can work in tandem with the body's endocannabinoid system to provide better health.

# THC and Health

As we said, the molecules that bind with the compounds in marijuana are receptors called CB1 and CB2. CB1 is mostly found in the brain—in fact, there are ten times as many CB1 receptors in the brain as there are opioid receptors responsible for the effects of morphine. THC causes the CB1 receptors to "over-activate," causing all kinds of psychological effects. Since everyone's body is different, everyone's "high" when using marijuana is different, as well. While some people experience euphoria and relaxation, others can feel anxious or paranoid.

And THC doesn't only affect the brain—it also binds to receptors in other areas of the body, like the CB2 receptors that are found on the cells of the immune system. When THC binds with these receptors, it can have an anti-inflammatory effect, which is one of the reasons the drug is gaining popularity as a medicinal remedy. THC can also stimulate the release of the hormone ghrelin—also known as "the hunger hormone"—which gives marijuana its notorious reputation for causing "the munchies."

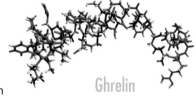

Ghrelin

Moreover, THC's anti-inflammatory properties have made it an increasingly popular therapeutic treatment for a host of ailments, like autoimmune disorders and multiple sclerosis. Researchers have also started to investigate the chemical's effects on cancer cells, with some promising results: THC has been shown to shrink cancer tumors in laboratory animals and prevent cancer from metastasizing.

Not only that, but the chemical's ability to increase dopamine is just like that of opioids—but THC is much safer and far less addictive. Couple that with its anti-inflammatory properties, and it's easy to see why one of THC's most popular medicinal uses is as a pain reliever.

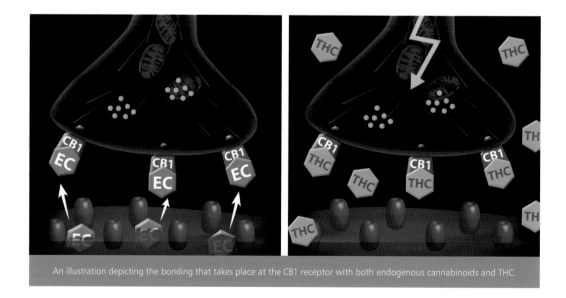

An illustration depicting the bonding that takes place at the CB1 receptor with both endogenous cannabinoids and THC.

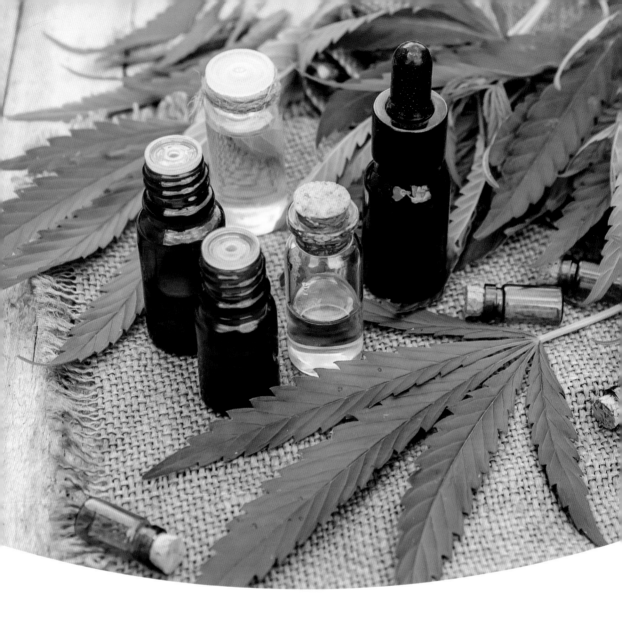

# The Benefits of CBD

As we've seen, THC binds with molecules in the brain's endocannabinoid system in order to produce its effects. While THC is the most talked-about cannabinoid in marijuana, because of its ability to cause a "high" and its medicinal properties, it is not the only one with benefits. Many of these compounds have yet to be studied in detail, and have tongue-twister names like cannabigerol, cannabinol, and cannabichromene. But another compound—cannabidiol, or CBD—is making headlines with its medicinal abilities, and some scientists think it could revolutionize medicine as we know it.

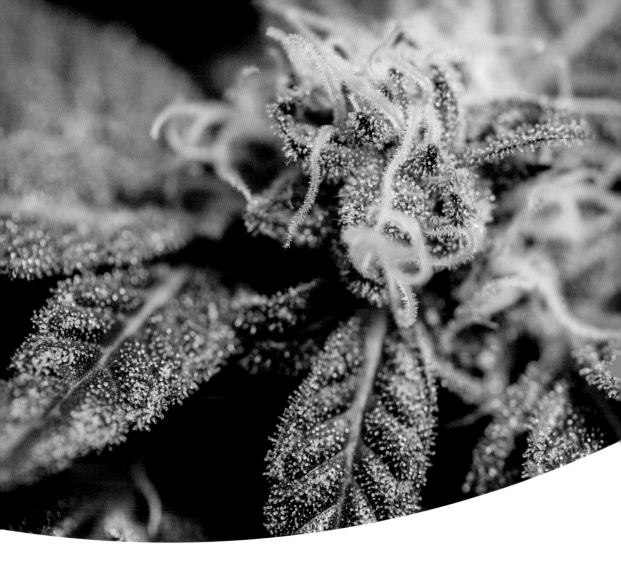

# Sourcing and Accessing CBD

Unlike THC, CBD is not psychoactive—meaning it can't give you the "high" associated with THC. This is an important attribute, as it is the THC in marijuana—not the other compounds—that is considered illegal in some states. So when CBD is isolated on its own, it can work its way around the legal issues that entangle THC.

Products containing CBD can easily be purchased in many stores or online. In fact, even the DEA has stated that curbing the use of CBD is not a priority. Still, the legality of marijuana in each state dictates where the CBD sold in that state comes from. If there are no medical cannabis laws in a state, CBD usually comes from low-to-no-THC hemp plants. But in states with medical cannabis laws, CBD can come from marijuana plants and, in some cases, can contain up to five percent THC.

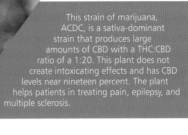

# The CBD Effect

One of the most promising effects CBD seems to have is as an anticonvulsant. Studies have shown that the compound works to prevent seizures and could be a great therapy for epilepsy. It has also been shown to have a "neuroprotective effect" which can prevent and treat neurological diseases like Alzheimer's, multiple sclerosis, and Parkinson's. Like THC, CBD has been shown to be a pain reliever, and it can also work together with morphine to counteract the opioid's side effects. CBD may slow the progression of cancer cells, reduce inflammation, and may help to treat mood disorders.

In addition to all of these, CBD provides one more benefit for those who choose to use marijuana recreationally: The compound actually acts as a counterweight to the psychoactive properties of THC, helping to reduce negative THC side-effects. For this reason, many cannabis users look for marijuana strains with a one to one THC/ CBD ratio.

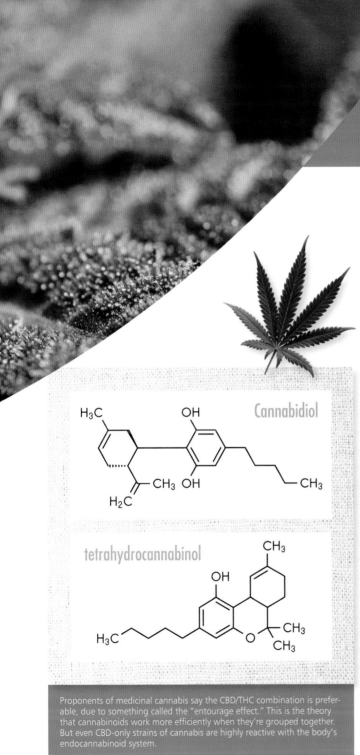

Proponents of medicinal cannabis say the CBD/THC combination is preferable, due to something called the "entourage effect." This is the theory that cannabinoids work more efficiently when they're grouped together. But even CBD-only strains of cannabis are highly reactive with the body's endocannabinoid system.

# Beyond THC and CBD

As mentioned, there are dozen—possibly upwards of a hundred—cannabinoids found in the marijuana plant. Some of these compounds haven't even been identified yet, and the restrictions on studying the plant have meant that discoveries have been slow. But scientists have isolated a few other cannabinoids and found that many of them have some unique benefits. These are just a handful of the cannabinoids found in marijuana. With so many benefits already discovered, it seems logical that more research and study needs to be allowed on the marijuana plant. Who knows what other medicinal secrets could be unlocked?

Cannabigerol

Cannabigerol, or CBG, is one such compound. Like CBD, this compound is not psychoactive, but CBG is sort of a "stem cell" for other cannabinoids, and can eventually turn into THC or CBD. On its own, it has anti-anxiety and muscle relaxing effects, and studies have shown that it works as an anti-inflammatory.

Cannabichromene, or CBC, is another compound found in cannabis. It is also not psychoactive, making it another promising cannabinoid for the future of medicine. CBC is even better at treating anxiety than CBD, and the effects last longer because the compound stays in the bloodstream for a long time. It's also been found to be anti-inflammatory, anti-bacterial, and anti-fungal. Amazingly, a University of Mississippi study even discovered that CBC helped to promote brain growth.

Cannabichromene

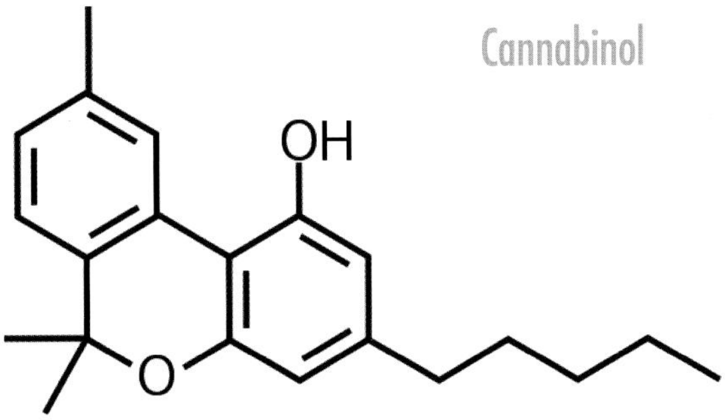

Cannabinol

Another cannabinoid in marijuana is cannabinol, or CBN. Although CBN is not considered psychoactive, it can have a very strong sedative effect. CBN forms when THC reacts with oxygen, so the longer cannabis is exposed to air, the more CBN it will contain. Because of its ability to cause drowsiness, CBN shows promise for treating insomnia and nerve pain.

Similar to THC is the cannabinoid tetrahydrocannabivarin, or THCV. And just like THC, THCV is also psychoactive. But unlike THC, THCV actually suppresses appetite rather than stimulates it. Because of this property, THCV is being studied as a possible weight-loss drug. It's also been shown to reduce the tremors that result from Parkinson's disease.

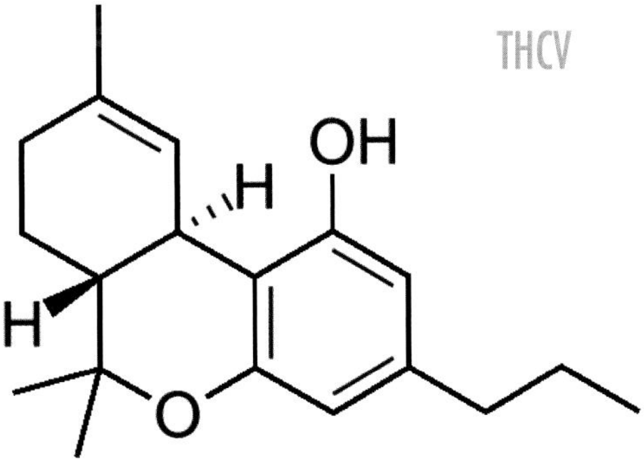

THCV

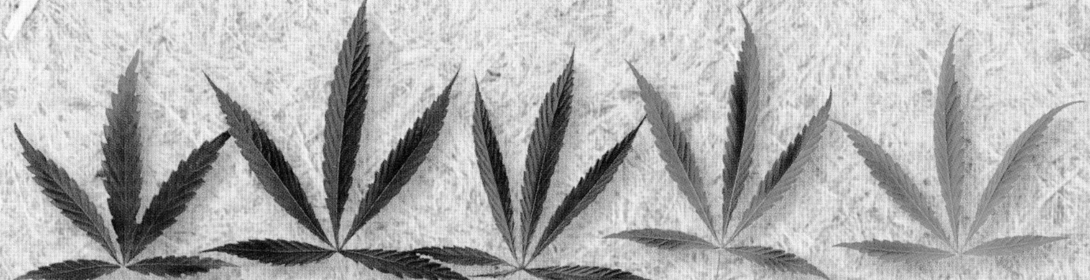

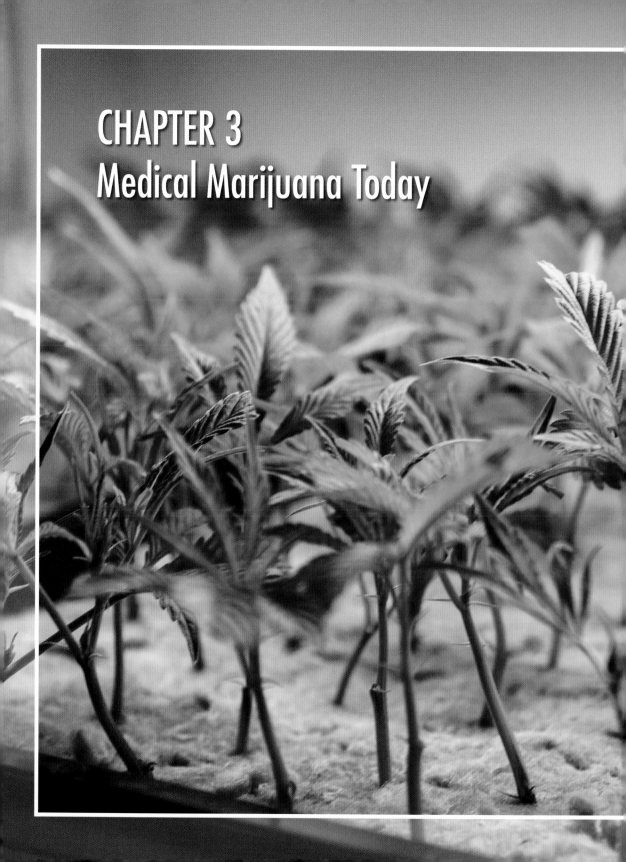

# CHAPTER 3
# Medical Marijuana Today

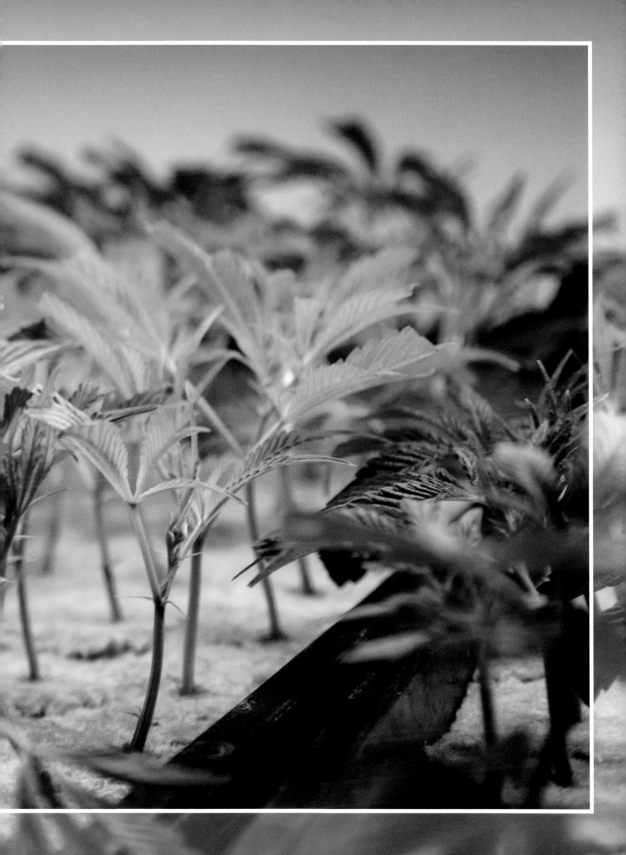

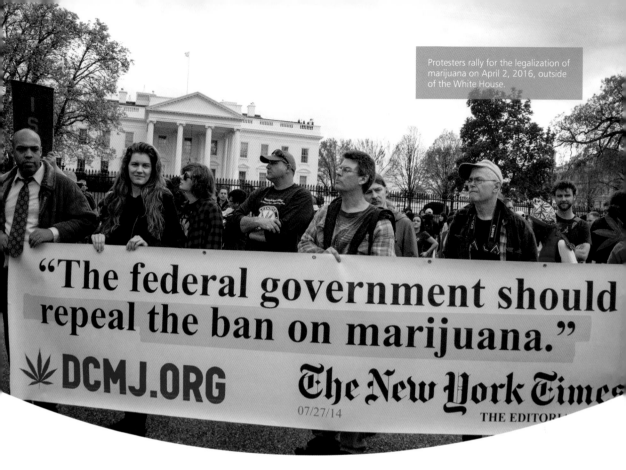

"The federal government should repeal the ban on marijuana."

DCMJ.ORG      The New York Times
07/27/14
THE EDITORI

# Cannabis and the Drug War

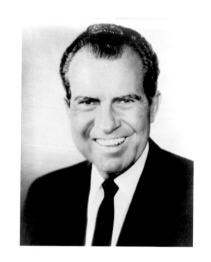

In 1970, President Richard Nixon signed the Controlled Substances Act into law, which established a federal drug policy. Recreational drug use had steadily climbed throughout the 1960s, and by the end of the decade nearly half of Americans believed that drug abuse was a serious problem in the country. Nixon proclaimed it "public enemy number one," and by June 1971 the president had officially declared a "War on Drugs."

As part of his strategy, Nixon increased federal funding for drug-control agencies and enacted strict penalties for drug offenses, including fines and mandatory prison time. In 1973, Nixon created the Drug Enforcement Administration (DEA), which consisted of 1,470 agents running on a budget of $75 million.

# Just Say No

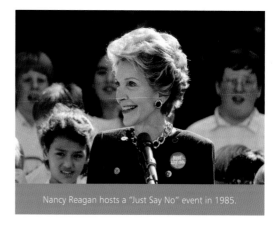

After Nixon left office, the War on Drugs calmed down a bit, with eleven states even passing laws to decriminalize marijuana. But in the 1980s, the conflict began anew, with Nancy Reagan's "Just Say No" campaign and a refocus on penalizing nonviolent drug crime. People began criticizing drug laws, with some believing they unfairly targeted people of color.

Nancy Reagan hosts a "Just Say No" event in 1985.

Interestingly, in the early 1980s less than six percent of Americans felt that drug abuse was a major issue in the country; but by the end of the decade—after years of hearing the "Just Say No" slogan—that number had climbed to sixty-four percent. Is it possible that an anti-drug campaign actually caused anti-drug hysteria?

Although anti-drug sentiment began declining by the 1990s, the stigma surrounding marijuana use remained. President Bill Clinton once famously said that he tried marijuana in his younger days, but "didn't inhale." There may have been few people who actually believed his claim, but whether true or not, it's easy to understand why the leader of the country would deny using the substance. But a couple decades later, President Barack Obama had a different answer when asked about his drug use: "When I was a kid, I inhaled frequently. That was the point," he said. Obama's candid statement echoed the changing attitudes toward cannabis in the twenty-first century—attitudes that have led to more and more states jumping on the legalization bandwagon.

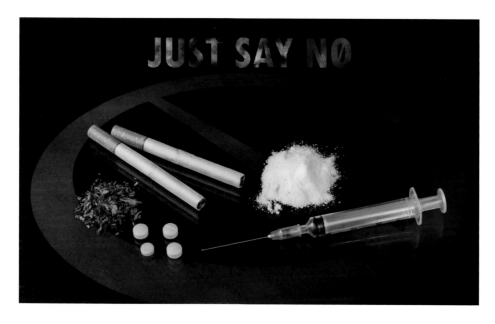

# Excessive Mass Incarceration

And yet, more than 700,000 people are still arrested for marijuana offenses every year. Decades after its inception, the DEA now employs 5,000 agents and has a budget that exceeds an astounding $2 billion. But after so much money has been spent and so many people arrested, Americans still frequently use marijuana. In fact, in 1969, just before the War on Drugs began, only four percent of Americans had experimented with the drug. But today, that number stands at thirty-eight percent. Clearly, the expensive "War on Drugs" has been a failure.

# Perceived Risk of Marijuana Use

A 2016 report on data collected between 2012 and 2014 shows that there are great regional differences in perceived risk of monthly marijuana use. (See the map to the right.) The study concludes that an annual average of nearly 75 million people in the U.S. believe that there is a large risk of harm from monthly marijuana smoking. That averages to about two out of every seven people, or about twenty-eight percent of the population in the U.S. These perceptions are largely held in the South, with sixteen of the highest percentage areas being found in the region. The sixteen lowest percentage areas were found along the Eastern Seaboard and the West Coast.

# The State of Legalization Today

As of 2018, thirty states and the District of Columbia have laws that make medical marijuana legal. These states include Alaska, Arizona, Arkansas, California, Colorado, Connecticut, Delaware, Florida, Hawaii, Illinois, Louisiana, Maine, Maryland, Massachusetts, Michigan, Minnesota, Montana, Nevada, New Hampshire, New Jersey, New Mexico, New York, North Dakota, Ohio, Oregon, Pennsylvania, Rhode Island, Vermont, Washington, and West Virginia. All of these states require proof of residency to acquire cannabis, to prevent out-of-state visitors from taking advantage of the system.

Each state also provides medical marijuana only for certain medical conditions (sorry, no marijuana for the common cold!), and several states do not allow the drug to be smoked.

Another sixteen states have legalized medicinal cannabis with low THC amounts or for patients with specific conditions.

Four states have no laws on the books that legalize marijuana in any form: Idaho, Kansas, Nebraska, and South Dakota. In these states, getting caught with even a small amount of cannabis could result in a hefty penalty.

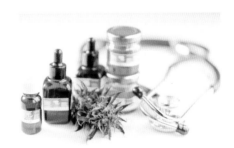

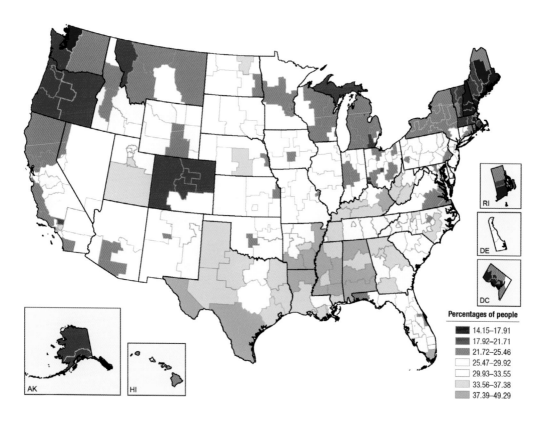

**Percentages of people**

- 14.15–17.91
- 17.92–21.71
- 21.72–25.46
- 25.47–29.92
- 29.93–33.55
- 33.56–37.38
- 37.39–49.29

RI

DE

DC

AK

HI

# Federal vs. State

Every year, more states vote to legalize marijuana, either for recreational or medicinal use. This is great news for proponents of the drug, but there's one caveat: federally, the drug remains illegal. This means that even if you are follow-ing state law when you buy or consume marijuana, you are still breaking federal law. Technically, you could even be charged with a federal crime. And federal law enforcement could po-tentially shut down cannabis-based businesses in states where such busi-nesses are legal.

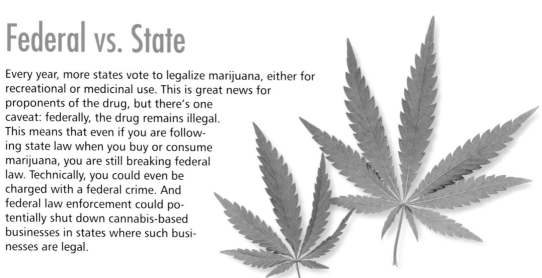

# Federal Hurdles and Roadblocks

This disconnect between state and federal laws has other ramifications, as well. For instance, many businesses that sell marijuana are cash-only establishments, because banks are wary about working with businesses that are breaking federal law. And a nervous bank is unlikely to make a loan to such a business. Cannabis-based businesses also can't file for certain tax deductions, thanks to section 280E of the federal tax code, which was originally aimed at illegal drug dealers. This means that a marijuana business can't deduct expenses like advertising, transportation, or rent, resulting in outlandish income tax rates that can exceed ninety percent. These roadblocks add up to a very expensive endeavor–obviously much more than a conventional business.

And those aren't the only hurdles faced by state-legal marijuana establishments. For instance, federal laws prohibit federally controlled water from being used for illegal marijuana farms—and since the drug is still illegal as far as the federal government is concerned, that includes farms in states where marijuana has been legalized. Marijuana farmers work around this by drilling wells or tapping into a city's water supply, but it's just one more inconvenience they must endure in order to run their business.

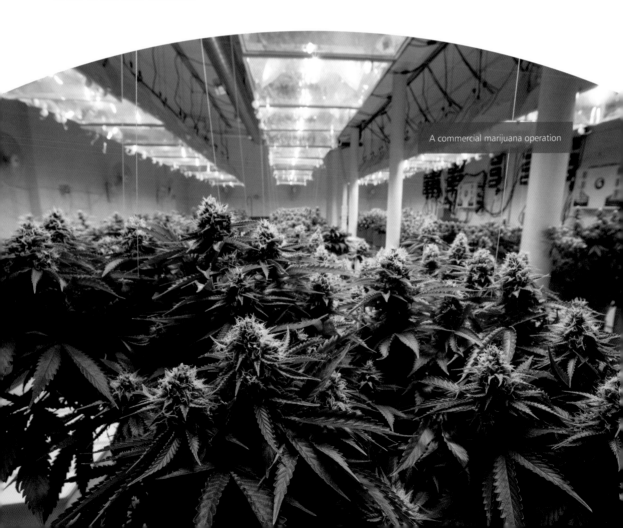

A commercial marijuana operation

Perhaps worst of all, the DEA is allowed to conduct raids on marijuana establishments, even in states where the drug is legal and the proprietors follow all state laws. Occasionally these raids are justifiable: there have been cases where owners of cannabis-based businesses have participated in money laundering or have even partnered with drug cartels. Others may have state-legal businesses but grow marijuana to illegally ship over the border into states where the drug is still illegal. But many DEA raids hit businesses that comply with all state laws, adding one more worry to the list of complications that owners of marijuana enterprises face.

Federal laws can also pose a problem for those who aren't engaged in selling the drug, but simply wish to use marijuana now and then, whether for recreation or for medical reasons. Since marijuana is still federally illegal, employers in any state—even those with legalization laws—can prohibit use of the drug as a condition of employment. The same holds true for renters: landlords can prohibit residents from using the substance, even in states where it is legal.

Because of the threat of a federal-government crackdown in states where marijuana is now medicinally and recreationally available, doctors may not prescribe medical marijuana without violating federal law and risking prosecution or losing their license. They may, however, recommend the therapy to a patient, but it's up to the patient to proceed from there.

# Schedule I and Studies

When the Controlled Substances Act was signed into law back in 1970, it established five different classifications—called "Schedules"—to help lawmakers and the medical industry decide how best to handle specific drugs. According to the DEA, drugs are assigned a Schedule "depending upon the drug's acceptable medical use and the drug's abuse or dependency potential." Drugs that are considered Schedule I are said to have a high risk for abuse and low potential for medicinal value; conversely, Schedule V drugs have a low risk for abuse and are commonly used as medicine.

Schedule I drugs include heroin, lysergic acid diethylamide (commonly known as LSD), ecstasy, peyote, and so-called "magic" mushrooms. Oh, and there's one more drug that joins the Schedule I list: Marijuana.

If you think it seems like a bit of overkill to place marijuana in the same category as heroin and LSD (and to place it in a higher category than cocaine and methamphetamine, which are classified as Schedule 2 drugs!) you're definitely not alone.

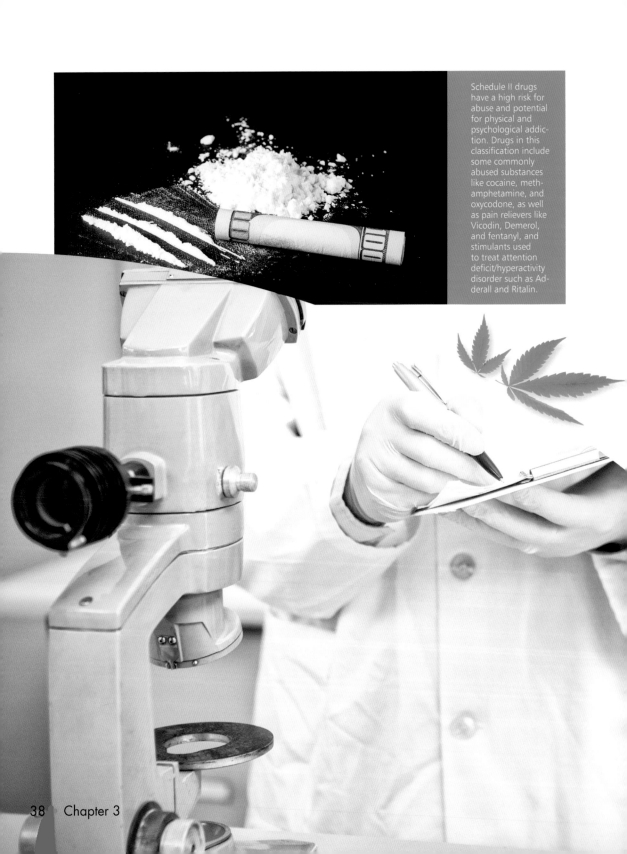

Schedule II drugs have a high risk for abuse and potential for physical and psychological addiction. Drugs in this classification include some commonly abused substances like cocaine, methamphetamine, and oxycodone, as well as pain relievers like Vicodin, Demerol, and fentanyl, and stimulants used to treat attention deficit/hyperactivity disorder such as Adderall and Ritalin.

The only reason cannabis remains a Schedule I drug is because there is insufficient scientific proof of its medical benefit. With thousands of years of anecdotal evidence and modern users who swear by its effectiveness, you would think that cannabis would at least be given a chance to prove itself.

But herein lies the problem: in order for marijuana to be rescheduled, it needs to be scientifically studied in controlled environments on a large scale, to collect enough evidence to prove its medical worth. But in order to conduct studies, researchers must get the approval of the DEA, which restricts how much marijuana can be researched. The very agency which requires scientific proof to reschedule a drug is restricting the study of that drug—so poor cannabis remains stuck at Schedule I.

But there is hope: the federal government has recently started easing some of the restrictions against studying marijuana, allowing researchers more access to the plant and enabling them to conduct larger studies. This could provide the proof of medicinal benefit needed to move the drug from Schedule I to Schedule II, although it wouldn't necessarily guarantee legal access for all.

# Marijuana vs. Opioid Use

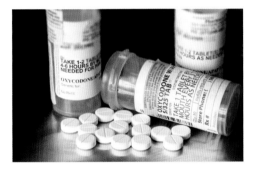

One promising fact is that in states that have legalized medical marijuana, opioid use is already dropping. A study published in *JAMA: The Journal of the American Medical Association* in May 2018 found that among those who use Medicare, opioid use dropped fourteen percent in states with access to medical marijuana. This is an estimated reduction of 3.7 million daily doses of opioids. While the study isn't necessarily definitive proof, as it shows only a correlation between lower opioid use and legal medical marijuana states, the two do seem to be connected: Prescriptions for medications to treat anxiety, nausea, and seizures (all of which marijuana has been shown to help) also dropped, whereas prescriptions for blood thinners (which cannot be replaced with marijuana) remained the same in these states. And since marijuana is far less addictive than opioids and does not cause overdoses, it could help save some of the thousands of lives lost to opioid overdoses every year. This is not to say that marijuana is without risks—all drugs have the potential to be abused—but the research clearly shows that medicinal cannabis could be a viable alternative to the frightening opioid epidemic in this country.

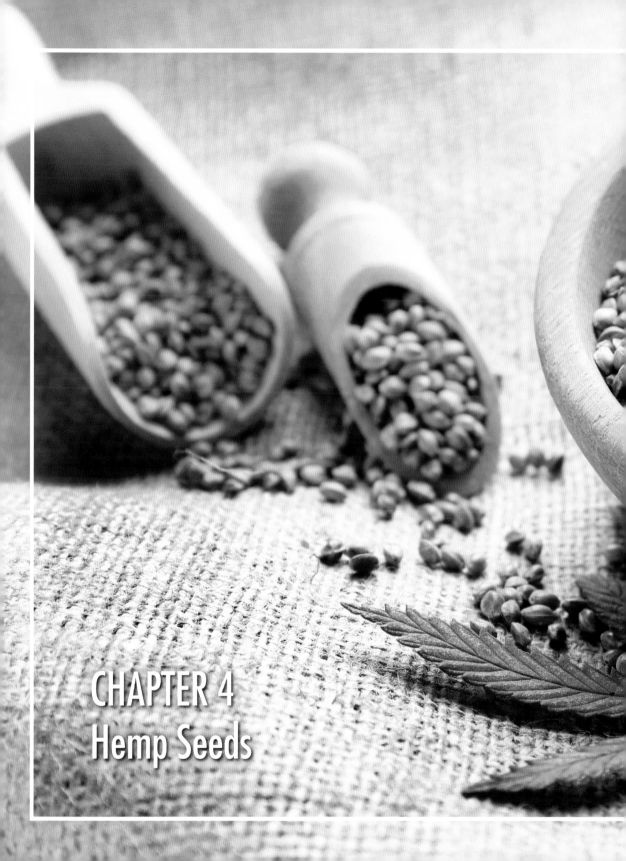

CHAPTER 4
Hemp Seeds

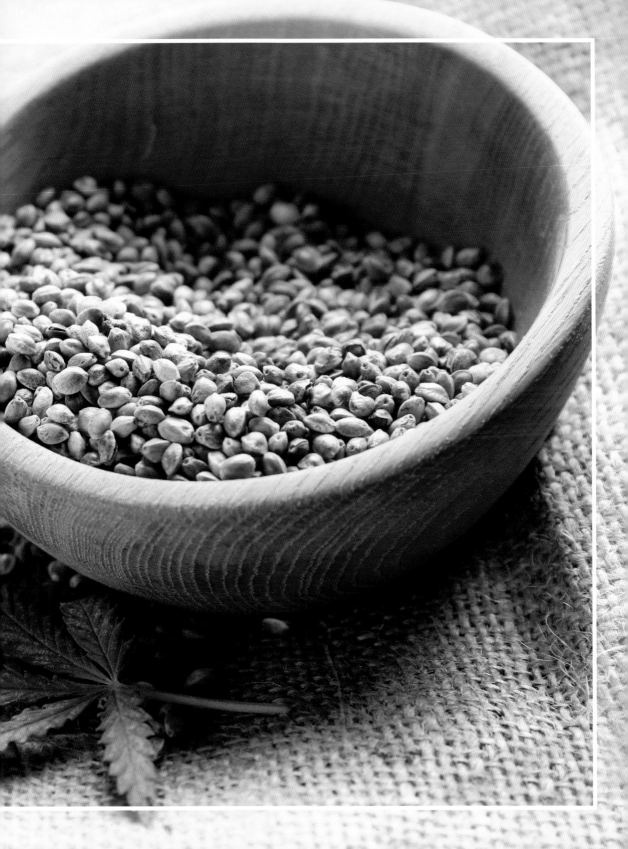

# Hemp Seeds and Health

Among the many products made from the *Cannabis sativa* plant are hemp seeds, and many nutritionists believe these seeds provide various health benefits. The small, brown seeds contain protein, fiber, and healthful fatty acids. They also contain antioxidants, which some believe help prevent or slow down various illnesses.

It's important to note that though the hemp and marijuana both come from the Cannabis plant, they are completely different. Hemp is grown specifically to create fiber, oil, and seeds.

Eating hemp seeds doesn't alter the mind because the seeds contain little if any of the specific THC chemical in the plant that produces a feeling of being high. Hemp seeds also contain a negligible amount of CBD, a compound in the cannabis plant that's different from THC.

Oils made from hemp seed are not the same as oils made from the entire hemp plant, which contains high concentrations of CBD, touted for health benefits. This book will discuss CBD oils and other products in great length. But this section focuses solely on hemp seeds.

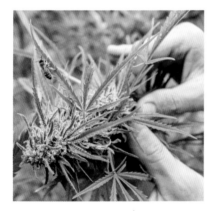

# From Plant to Seed

Harvesting hemp seeds from the Cannabis plant involves choosing the time at which the most amount of mature seeds is available. That's usually when the plant has been growing for about four months. Lower seeds on the plant mature more quickly than those near the top.

Farmers harvest hemp seed with a combine tractor. They remove leaves, immature seeds, and other unwanted products before storing the seed in grain bins.

Three tablespoons of hemp seeds contain 116 calories and provides 9.47 grams of protein, 2.6 grams of carbohydrates and 1.2 grams of fat and 14.62 grams of total fatty acids, most of which are unsaturated, according to the United States Department of Agriculture.

# Health Benefits

Vegetarians eat hemp seeds because they contain all of the essential amino acids needed for a complete protein. Humans need to absorb some of these amino acids through food because the body doesn't produce all of them. Vegetarians are cautioned, however, not to use hemp seeds as their sole source of protein.

Hemp seeds also contain healthful fatty acids, specifically Omega 3s, which humans often don't get enough of. Omega 3s are linked to maintaining a healthy heart and reducing acne as well as other skin conditions.

Hemp seeds contain no trans fats and are low in saturated fats.

Hemp seeds also provide both soluble and insoluble fiber, especially when the outer hull or shell is kept intact. A high fiber diet can help maintain a healthy weight, reduce cholesterol, and keep blood sugar levels stable.

Ingesting hemp seeds has been said to reduce symptoms of premenstrual syndrome and menopause and may reduce your risk of heart disease. Some studies show eating hemp seeds could also aid in digestion and help with skin disorders.

Overall, hemp seeds contain vitamin B and E, magnesium, phosphorous, potassium, iron and zinc, all necessary for good health.

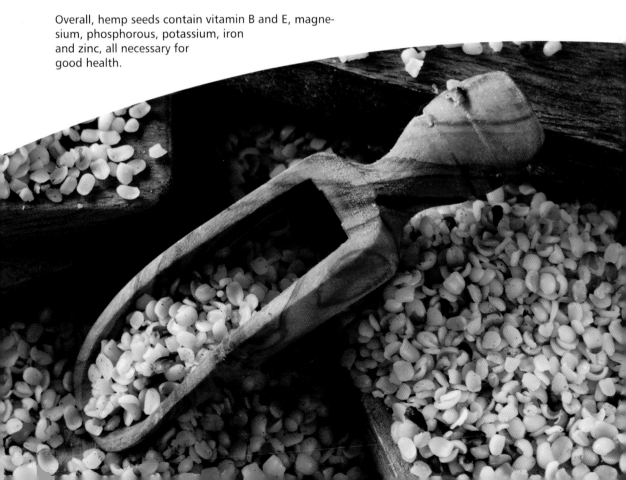

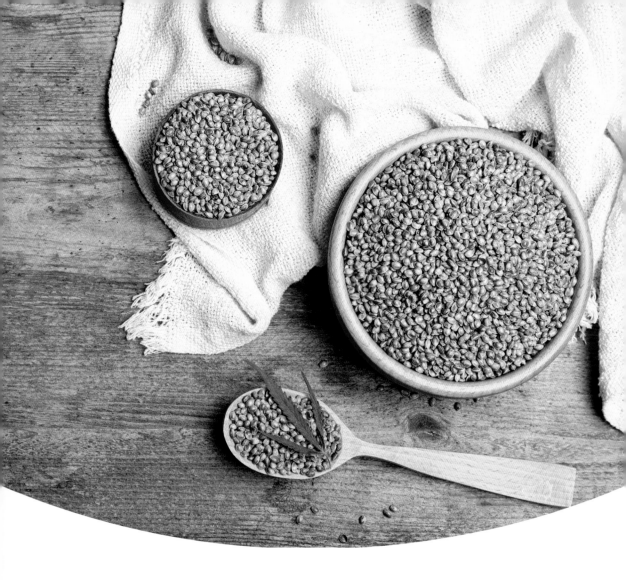

# Choosing Hemp Seeds

Before purchasing hemp seed, read the labels and make sure it's thoroughly cleaned and contains no contaminants. Most reports say the highest quality hemp seed can be obtained from Canada. Choosing hemp seed made from China is discouraged. You can buy hemp seeds either hulled or un-hulled.

High-quality hemp seeds are said to taste soft and nutty; if they taste bitter, don't use them. When purchasing hemp seed online, read the reviews to help decide what's best for you, and what might be a good product. If purchasing at a store, ask the owner questions about its origin, uses, and different ways it's packaged. Also consider purchasing a hemp cookbook to expand ways to use the seeds.

# Preparation and Use

Before using, wash hemp seeds by soaking them in water, then draining in a colander. You can toss raw hemp seeds onto oatmeal, yogurt, cereal, and salads or add to pancake batter or scrambled eggs or omelets while cooking. Use hemp seed in homemade granola or mix it in with a smoothie. To create hemp seed milk, combine 3 cups of water, 1 cup of hemp seed, and a sweetener such as honey if you'd like.

Hemp seed also can be used as a substitute for bread crumbs on various meats such as chicken. Dip chicken into some milk and beaten eggs, then coat with the hemp seed, and bake in the oven.

Toasted hemp seeds are also available and can be eaten as a snack. Or toast your own by putting them in a wok and stirring under medium heat. Be careful not to burn them; otherwise, the flavor will turn bitter. The seeds are well toasted when they begin to pop like popcorn.

You can also create your own hemp flour by toasting hemp seeds, then grinding them in a coffee grinder. Purchasing hemp flour might be an easier choice. Hemp flour is gluten-free, but it does have a strong flavor, so adding it to other flours with a ratio of about 1:5 is recommended. It usually can last about six months if kept cool and in an airtight container.

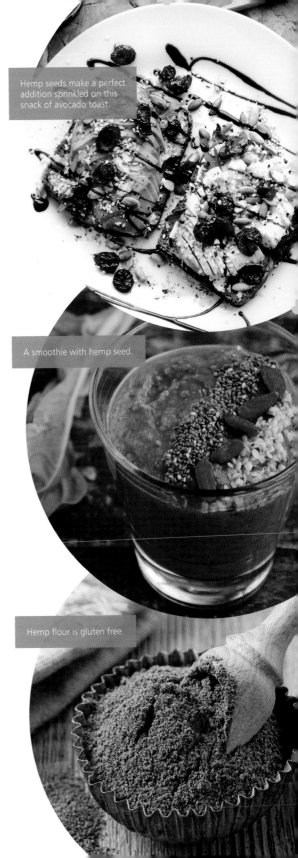

Hemp seeds make a perfect addition sprinkled on this snack of avocado toast.

A smoothie with hemp seed.

Hemp flour is gluten free.

Hemp seed oil.

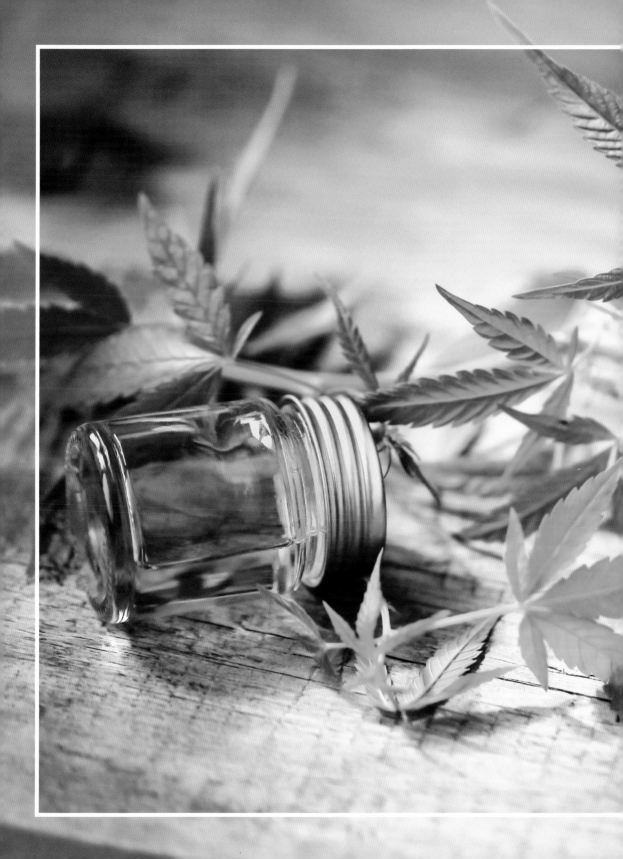

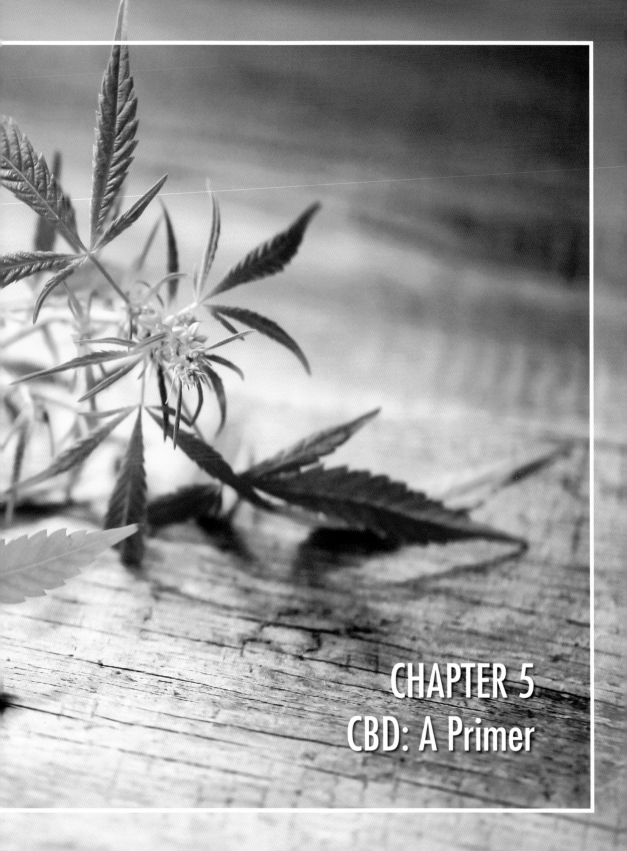

# CHAPTER 5
# CBD: A Primer

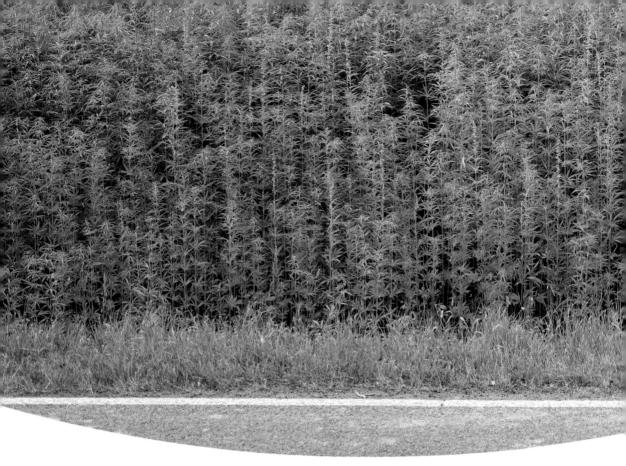

# What's What:
# CBD Oil, Hemp Oil, and Cannabidiol

Many products are made from various strains of the *Cannabis sativa* plant and contain differing amounts of the most prevalent chemicals in the plant, Tetrahydrocannabinol, or THC, and cannabidiol, or CBD. Those containing high concentrates of THC, the chemical that creates a high or euphoric feeling along with mood-altering and behavioral changes, come from the marijuana plant, *Cannabis sativa*. Products including oils and isolates with a high amount of CBD, which doesn't produce a high, and a minimal to no amount of THC come from industrial hemp, which is a subspecies of *Cannabis sativa*.

As of October 2018, medical marijuana was legal in some form in 30 states, and nine states and the District of Columbia allow recreational marijuana use, according to CNN. CBD oil made from hemp is legal to consume in many countries and most of the United States, according to CBD product manufacturers.

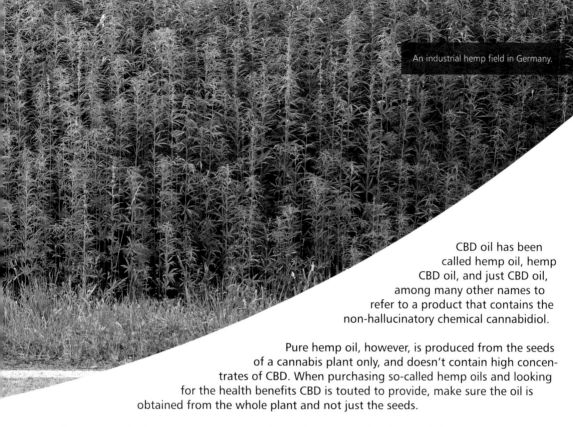

CBD oil has been called hemp oil, hemp CBD oil, and just CBD oil, among many other names to refer to a product that contains the non-hallucinatory chemical cannabidiol.

Pure hemp oil, however, is produced from the seeds of a cannabis plant only, and doesn't contain high concentrates of CBD. When purchasing so-called hemp oils and looking for the health benefits CBD is touted to provide, make sure the oil is obtained from the whole plant and not just the seeds.

Products made from CBD oil can be purchased in stores and online, and they have been touted as a health benefit for many conditions including depression, insomnia, cancer, substance abuse, anxiety, skin disease, diabetes, heart disease and other ailments. Also, note that the FDA approved in late 2018 the first drug made from CBD oil to treat a rare form of epilepsy. (See more on that in the section on the future of CBD oil that begins on page 81.)

As of May 2018, CBD was legal in 44 states. Six states considered CBD illegal: South Dakota, Idaho, Kansas, Nebraska, Indiana, and West Virginia. In September 2018, a North South Dakota store was told it could no longer sell CBD oil because of a new law in the books.

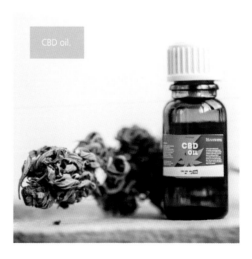

CBD oil.

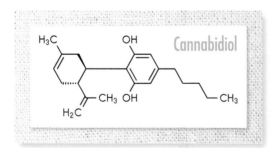

H₃C    OH    Cannabidiol

CH₃  OH                CH₃
H₂C

# Legality, the Farm Bill and the Hemp Act

Industrial hemp and marijuana look and are grown quite differently. Generally, hemp stalks are long, thin, and fibrous, while marijuana plants are not as tall and appear from a distance as being short, round bushes. The leaves on marijuana are broad; those on hemp are skinnier. Hemp can be grown as close as 4 inches apart, but medical cannabis needs to be grown much farther apart, perhaps up to 6 feet.

Industrial hemp was widely grown in the U.S. during the mid-1800s for fabric, wine, and paper. In 1937, industrial hemp was determined by law to be a narcotic drug and growing it in the U.S. was illegal.

The 2014 farm bill signed by President Barack Obama paved the way for the nationwide legal production of industrial hemp, from which CBD oil is made. Industrial hemp is defined as containing no more than 0.3 percent of THC.

The farm bill allows pilot programs and research on industrial hemp. States were given leeway to provide regulations about growing and researching industrial hemp. At least 39 states have instituted cultivation and production programs for industrial hemp.

The Hemp Farming Act of 2018 was introduced to make industrial hemp and all products including CBD oil and isolates made from it throughout the U.S. legal. As of this writing, the U.S. Senate passed the act, and it was awaiting approval from

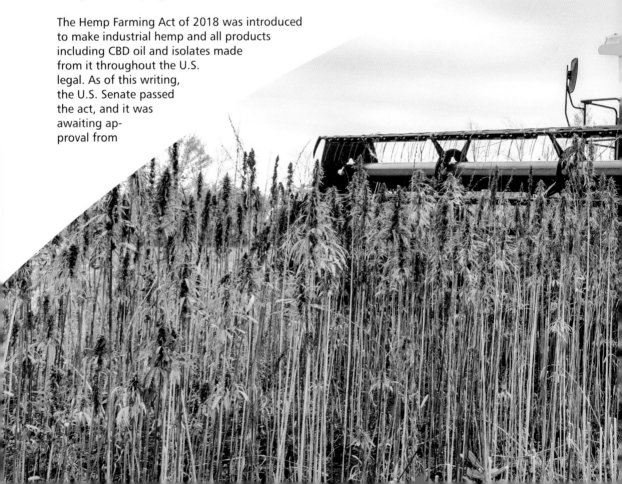

the House and a signature by the president, but hurdles remained. The act considers CBD oil made from industrial hemp a food supplement. In essence, the legislation would remove hemp—including hemp-derived CBD—from the Controlled Substances Act.

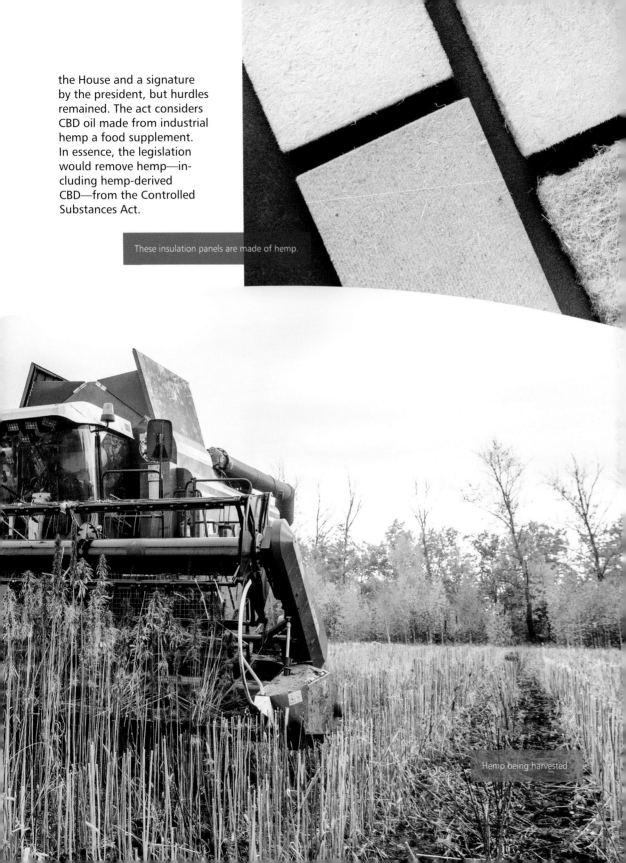

These insulation panels are made of hemp.

Hemp being harvested.

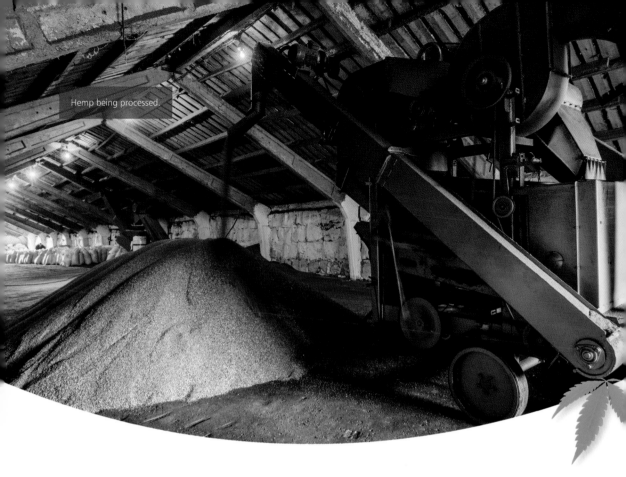

Hemp being processed.

# From State to State

State legislatures have addressed a variety of policies in their laws regarding CBD. These include the definition of hemp, licensing for growers, regulation of seeds, and more, according to the National Conference of State Legislatures. At least 41 states have passed legislation related to industrial hemp, such as defining hemp and removing barriers, and at least 39 states have allowed for hemp cultivation and production programs, according a conference report. In 2018, Alaska, Arizona, Kansas, Missouri, and Oklahoma passed legislation establishing hemp research and industrial hemp pilot programs.

States laws vary and can be quite complex. At least 38 states considered legislation related to industrial hemp in 2018. These bills ranged from clarifying existing laws to establishing new licensing requirements and programs.

Except for West Virginia, all states with industrial hemp definition statutes use the guidelines in which the product contains no more than 0.3 percent of THC. In West Virginia, as of this writing, industrial hemp is defined as having less than 1 percent of THC. Some states measure the THC concentration based on the plants' dry weight and others have passed laws stating an industrial hemp grower has to be licensed.

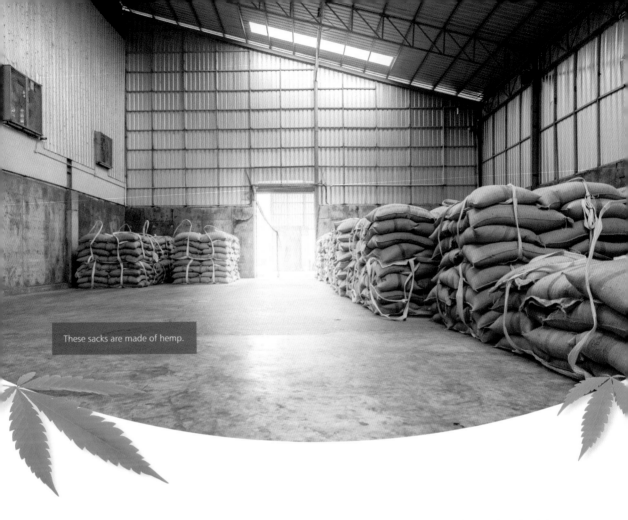

These sacks are made of hemp.

Some states have specific requirements on what industrial hemp seeds can be used and sold. For example, Oregon requires growers who sell seeds to register with the state department of agriculture. In Maine, the commissioner of agriculture, conservation, and forestry issues licenses to seed distributors if they obtain them from a certified source. In Hawaii, the board of agriculture certifies hemp seeds. Arizona allows commercial hemp production, processing, and manufacturing. Maine and South Carolina allow the growing of hemp for commercial purposes. In Virginia, separate licenses are required for commercial growers and for those working in research programs. In some states, higher learning institutions cultivating industrial hemp are required to provide periodic reports. Businesses in states that allow for commercial cultivation sometimes grow, manufacture, and sell their own CBD products online.

This is an important issue to states and their agricultural practices because industrial hemp can be used to manufacture a wide variety of products including fibers, textiles, paper, construction and insulation materials, cosmetic products, animal feed, food, and beverages. The plant is estimated to be used in more than 25,000 products, according to the National Conference of State Legislatures.

# CBD Oil's Growing Popularity

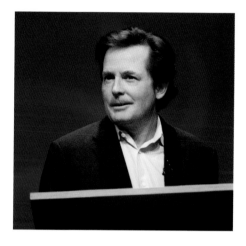

People are turning to CBD oil hoping to get the same benefits of using marijuana with no chance of getting high, and to be compliant with the law. A number of celebrities tout the benefits of CBD beauty and health products. A model for Victoria's Secret has said she uses CBD oil to help her sleep at night. Jennifer Aniston has been quoted as saying she uses CBD oil to help with pain, stress, and anxiety. Mandy Moore has been said to use CBD balms on her feet to ease the pain from wearing high heels all day. Whoopi Goldberg has used a vaping pen with CBD oil to treat pain and stress. And Michael Fox is said to use CBD oil to reduce the symptoms of Parkinson's disease.

Sales for products made with CBD oils continue to skyrocket. The total U.S. consumer sales of CBD in the U.S. in 2014 was $1.8 million, according to Statistics Portal. The number has grown each year since, and estimates show in the year 2020 CBD consumer sales will total roughly $1.5 billion in the U.S. If the Hemp Farming Act of 2018 passes, some estimate that number could soar to $20 billion. In addition, another study conducted by the Brightfield Group says if the act passes, the market for hemp-derived CBD will be bigger than the market for legal pot, and that CBD sales could reach $22 billion by 2022.

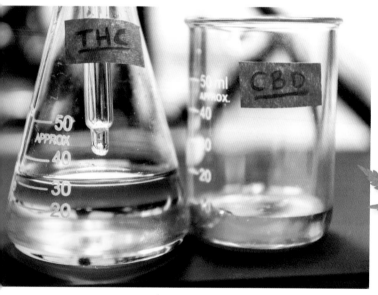

Before describing the various forms in which hemp CBD can be purchased, it might be useful to learn how it is made, and the difference between oils and isolates.

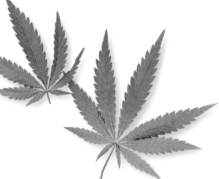

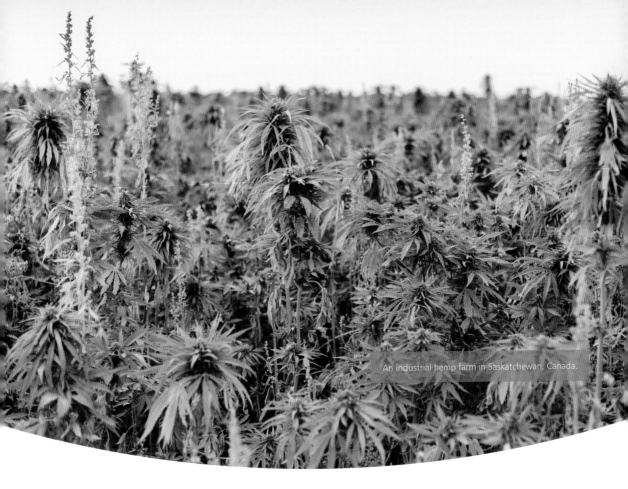

An industrial hemp farm in Saskatchewan, Canada.

# How CBD Oils and Isolates Are Made

Making CBD oil starts with choosing the right plant strain grown in proper conditions. Many industrial hemp growers opt to farm the plant organically—and in fact, the crop needs less water, pesticides, herbicides, and fertilizers compared with corn. Industrial hemp is considered a sustainable crop in the U.S., but as of now, there's no real way to designate whether it's been organically grown.

A variety of strains of industrial hemp are available—one of them is called Fedora 17 and is said to have one of the lowest THC contents among different strains. Another strain known as Charlotte's web is said to have a high CBD concentration and low THC concentration. Developed in 2011 through crossbreeding marijuana with industrial hemp, the Charlotte's web strain was nicknamed Hippie's disappointment, because it does not make the user high.

Industrial hemp is being grown legally on 26,000 acres in 19 states, according to a *Modern Farmer* article published in July 2018. Most of the industrial hemp used for CBD oil still comes from other countries such as Canada, but if the Hemp Farming Act of 2018 passes, making it legal to grow nationwide, that could change.

Hemp can be grown from seed, which has been difficult to find in the U.S., or propagated from tissue culture and then transferred into pots with soil in greenhouses and eventually outdoors.

A fairly easy way to make CBD oil from the hemp plant is by using a solvent such as ethanol, which extracts the cannabinoids from the plant. The solvent is then evaporated, leaving the CBD hemp oil behind. Ethanol is considered safe by the FDA and used as a food preservative, but there are some minuses to this technique. The method also extracts chlorophyll, which leaves the oil with a bitter flavor; filters can be used to remove the chlorophyll, but that might also remove some of the desirable chemicals touted to have health effects. Trying this at home is not recommended because it can be dangerous.

With the olive oil extraction method, the plant is heated to a certain temperature for a specific amount of time. Then the plant is placed into the olive oil and heated again. Companies rarely use this method because it yields small amounts of product and requires lots of labor hours.

A more advanced and the most common method used by companies involves using carbon dioxide, the same stuff used to put bubbles in your soda. It's considered safe and results in a purer product compared with the solvent method. Food companies have used carbon dioxide extraction method for years, for example, to remove caffeine from coffee or to create essential oils.

To produce CBD oils, carbon dioxide extraction involves using the dried and ground hemp plant. Manufactures either use a supercritical, subcritical, or mid-critical technique to extract the oil. All techniques require expensive equipment and trained chemists to do the work.

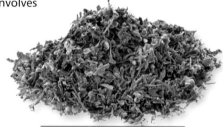

Dried hemp leaves and seeds.

The most common carbon dioxide extraction method is supercritical. The carbon dioxide held within a chamber is manipulated by dropping the temperature to below negative 69 degrees Fahrenheit and increasing pressure to more than 75 pounds per square inch.

The supercritical carbon dioxide then gets passed through the plant in an extractor. The carbon dioxide pulls the essential oils out of the plant, which get sent to a collection vessel. The result is a golden yellow, somewhat thick oil. The supercritical carbon dioxide gets turned back into a liquid and can be used for the next batch.

This method enables the carbon dioxide to act almost as if it were a gas and a liquid at the same time. Supercritical extraction also extracts the waxes, fats, and other substances from the plant, which can, according to some experts, enhance the quality of the product.

The subcritical extraction method involves lower temperatures and lower pressures, resulting in lighter oil. Some experts say the subcritical extraction is less likely to damage some of the good chemicals in the plant, but it might not extract fatty acids such as Omega 3. Some companies use a combination of both methods to extract CBD.

CBD extraction methods are evolving—and new ideas are coming forth involving the use of microwave and ultrasonic methods. A Canadian-based manufacturer has started using targeted radio microwaves that heat moisture within the plant, causing pressure to build and the desirable oils to seep out of the plant. The ultrasonic method, which is similar to the microwave method, is considered quick and environmentally friendly, but the cost to purchase the equipment is highly expensive.

Some experts prefer the whole plant extraction method because they believe it interacts better with the human endocannabinoid system. They call it the entourage effect, meaning the oil contains a full spectrum of chemicals from the hemp plant. As such, the product likely has more substances, which can be beneficial to the health.

Manufacturers are now touting isolates as a way to get the most potent form of CBD without any THC content.

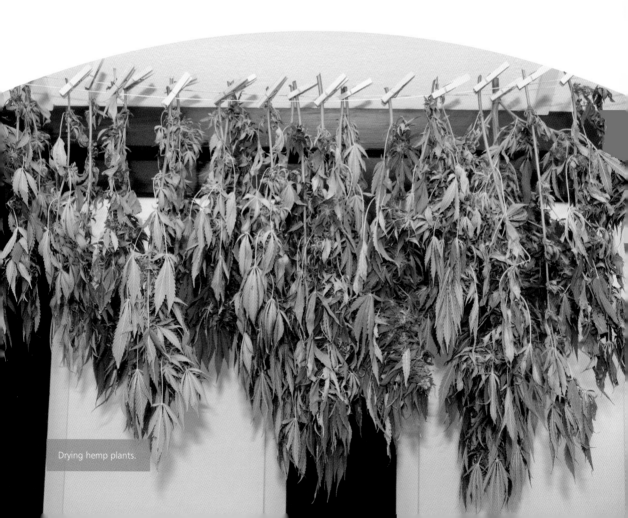

Drying hemp plants.

# Isolates Extraction

With isolates extraction, the result is a white powder or tiny, white crystals. You can purchase isolates in that form or in a carrier oil such as olive oil that has been infused with the isolates. Creating isolates begins with extracting the oil using one of the methods mentioned above. Chemists then use a separation or purification method to remove all plant materials and other chemicals besides the CBD. The resulting compound is then heated to create the isolates, a pure powder that contains 99 percent CBD. Scientists call it a single cannabinoid compound, meaning all the THC has been removed. Those who use isolated CBD should not test positive on a drug tests checking THC levels, according to manufacturers of the product.

One criticism of using pure isolates is that they contain none of the other beneficial cannabinoids found in CBD oil using the whole plant extraction method—and scientists are just beginning to study how various cannabinoids within the Cannabis plant might work together to enhance different health benefits.

With all these methods, the best products are those tested by independent labs to ensure they don't contain toxins, heavy metals, and other unwanted substances. The labs should also analyze the content and potency of the oil or isolates before selling it for formulation into consumer products.

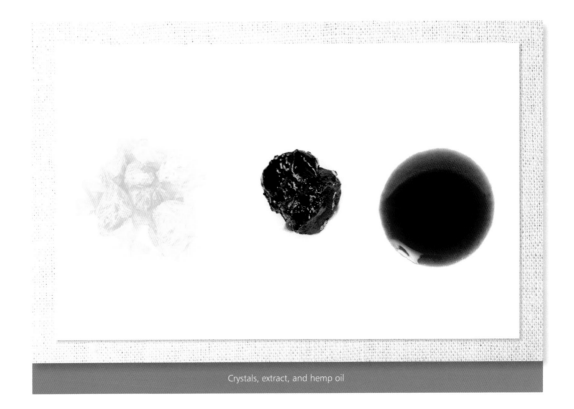

Crystals, extract, and hemp oil

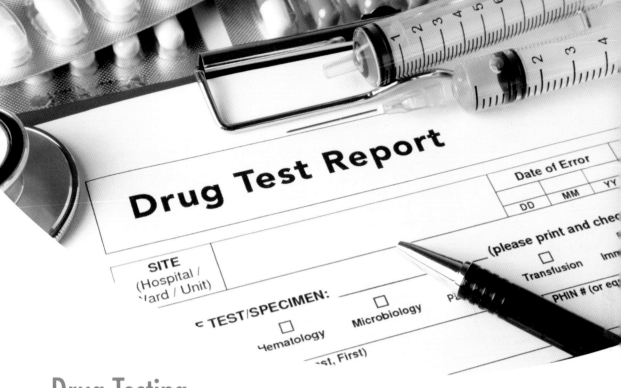

# Drug Testing

Employers who require urinalysis drug tests for their workers typically follow guidelines from agencies such as the Substance Abuse and Mental Health Services Administration. These agencies set guidelines for cut-off levels regarding the presence of THC, which is found in marijuana. The cut off is 50 nanograms per milliliter. If it's 50 or above, the test is positive. Then another more specific test is done to determine a final positive or negative.

If you use CBD oil, which can contain small traces of THC, can you test positive?

You'd have to have ingested very large amounts of CBD, but it's possible, and research shows that CBD stays in your system for about three to five days, even if its effects only last for several hours. Generally, if you're consuming more than 1,000 milligrams of CBD daily, it could produce a false positive on the drug test. Most CBD users ingest about 120 to 160 milligrams per day.

Something else to consider is the fact that the FDA doesn't regulate CBD oil products, and has warned consumers that not all claims by manufacturers regarding the amount of CBD contained in products are accurate. If a lot more is present than what's on the label, that could add to your THC levels.

If you want to make sure you're not ingesting even a trace of THC, you can use products made with CBD isolates. The process as well as the pluses and minuses of using isolates is described on the previous page.

The best way to insure you won't test positive on a marijuana drug test while taking hemp CBD oil is to purchase high-quality products, according to experts, but remember, there's always a chance you will test positive.

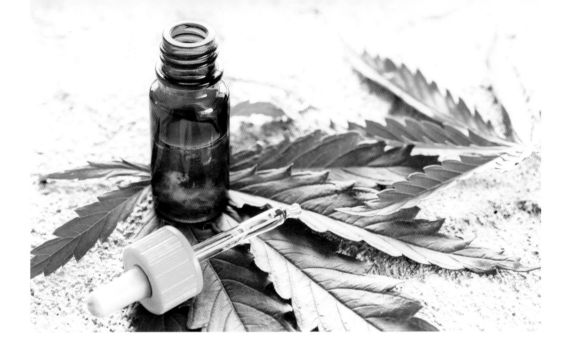

# CBD Oil Forms

Once you're ready to start using CBDs, you'll be bombarded with many forms in which to purchase it. These include concentrated oils, tinctures, sprays, balms, waxes, dabs, vapes, and isolated crystals, among others.

The two most popular ways include purchasing CBD oil either in a concentrate or in a tincture. CBD tinctures and CBD oils are taken orally—and sometimes the terms are used interchangeably. To make CBD oil into an ingestible concentrate, manufacturers add what's called a carrier oil, which is typically olive oil, vegetable oil, or hemp seed oil—note that this hemp seed oil is made solely from hemp seeds and is not the same as hemp CBD oil.

Typically, CBD oil is sold in a small bottle, usually with a dropper, and can be ingested orally or added to food. A few drops can be placed underneath the tongue, held there for about 90 seconds, and then swallowed.

Another common way to ingest CBD oil is through tinctures, which are generally infused with alcohol. Tinctures can be ingested the same as CBD oil concentrates: by placing a few drops beneath your tongue. You may find what are called flavored CBD oils on the market that are actually tinctures. As always, read the labels carefully.

CBD oil can also be delivered via oral sprays. For example, you can purchase a CBD oil full-spectrum peppermint spray, which delivers 1 mg of CBD every two sprays.

Rave, an online product reviewer, listed the top 20 CBD oils on the market in October 2018. The top 10 include Fab, cbdMD, Populum, CBDistillery, Pure Hemp Botanicals, Receptra Naturals, Canna Trading Co., MedTerra, Hemplucid and Palmetto Harmony. These companies sell oils and tinctures, flavored and unflavored.

# Vaporizer and Dab Pens

Another common way to use CBD is in a vaporizer pen. For that you'll need to purchase the pen as well as CBD vape liquids, which are less syrupy than CBD oils or tinctures. In fact, tinctures absolutely cannot be used with vaporizer pens, and hopefully that's indicated on the labels of pens for sale. To make sure you're purchasing the right product, read the label. It will often say CBD vaping oil, CBD juice, or CBD e-liquid. Some manufacturers might call it CBD vaping oil, when it really should be called CBD vape liquid. The most important thing to remember is that you cannot vape a CBD oil or tincture made to be taken under the tongue.

Vaping CBD liquid is said to get into your system even more quickly than ingesting concentrated oil. It, too, comes in a variety of flavors.

You'll have to purchase a vape pen, which comes with a tank, an atomizer, sensors, and a battery with a USB charger. These work together to heat the liquid and produce vapor. Read the instructions on how to insert batteries, fill the small tank with oil, and turn the product off and on. It can take several hours to charge the vape pen.

When the vape pen is on, insert it into your mouth and inhale. It's OK if you get it into your lungs, or you can hold it in your mouth for a while and then blow it out. Your body responds to the CBD much more quickly when vaping then ingesting. Experts recommend purchasing high-quality vape pens, because substandard ones could be harmful.

In addition, you need to be careful when purchasing CBD vape liquids. Some could contain harsh chemicals that were added when thinning the oil. Two of these are propylene glycol and polyethylene glycol—and they can break down into cancer-causing substances. A 2010 study found that inhaling propylene glycol could cause allergic reactions and potentially asthma.

Another type of pen you might see is called a dab pen, sometimes called a wax pen. It's used solely for inhaling dabs, which look like wax. You cannot use vape and dab pens interchangeably. Dab pens were created specifically for the marijuana user who wants to dab with high concentrates of THCs. Obviously that's not legal in many states. But you can purchase dabs that only contain CBDs. The wax is dabbed into a chamber or smeared across coils. Then you choose a temperature to heat the wax, typically three different settings. Then you put the pen in your mouth and inhale slowly. Use a dab pen that has glass or steel on the top of the mouthpiece, rather than plastic or rubber.

Be aware that when searching online, the terms vape pen and wax pen and dab pen can get confusing, so read all the product information before choosing.

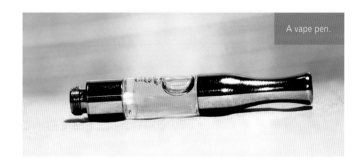
A vape pen.

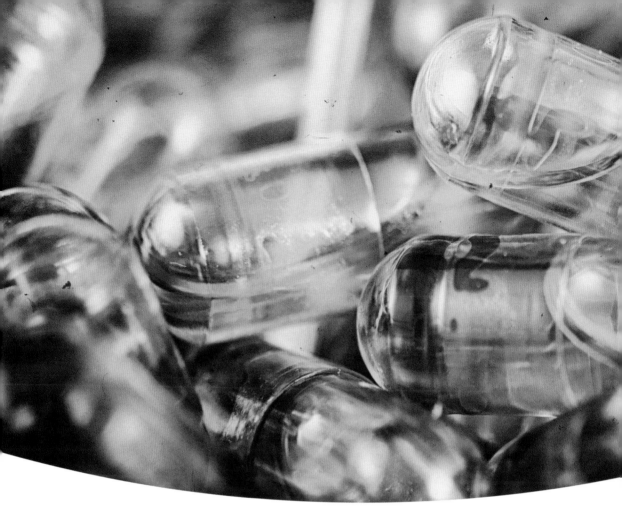

# Pills, Patches and Suppositories

CBD also can be purchased in gel capsules and other pill forms in various strengths. CBD gel capsules can be made from either full-spectrum or isolate CBD. They're easy to take and it's easier to know exactly how much dosage you're taking daily. Capsules are easy to swallow and you can include them with your vitamin or prescription daily regimens. If you want to adjust your dosage by just a few milligrams, you can try adding a drop of tincture or oil to your daily regimen along with the capsule and see how that works.

Another way to administer CBD is through a wearable patch. The patch typically delivers constant dosing for one to several days without having to remove it, and many are waterproof so you can take a shower or bath while wearing them. One pro of using a patch includes its time-release delivery, which doesn't enter the digestive tract. Some manufacturers tout their patches as being natural vitamin patches free of additives and preservatives.

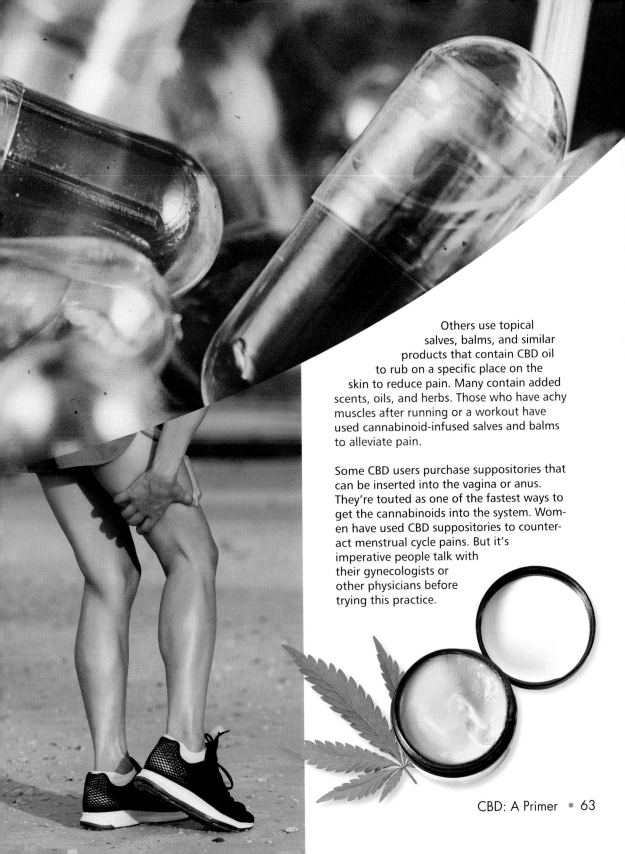

Others use topical salves, balms, and similar products that contain CBD oil to rub on a specific place on the skin to reduce pain. Many contain added scents, oils, and herbs. Those who have achy muscles after running or a workout have used cannabinoid-infused salves and balms to alleviate pain.

Some CBD users purchase suppositories that can be inserted into the vagina or anus. They're touted as one of the fastest ways to get the cannabinoids into the system. Women have used CBD suppositories to counteract menstrual cycle pains. But it's imperative people talk with their gynecologists or other physicians before trying this practice.

# Purchasing and Using Isolates

CBD isolates come in white powders that can be placed under the tongue just like CBD oil tinctures. They're tasteless, which is one reason some people prefer them over concentrated CBD oils or tinctures.

You can also make your own CBD-infused oils by adding isolates to oils such as palm, avocado, and coconut. Then add the oil to your smoothies, coffee, yogurt, honey, and other drinks and foods. The oil can also be massaged onto your muscles. Some people use the pure isolate with an oil of their choice instead of purchasing a balm or salve that might contain unwanted ingredients such as scents. CBD isolates also have been added to vape oil and wax pen products to boost the cannabinoid content. Sometimes CBD manufacturers also add terpenes to the CBD isolate to create what's called CBD shatter. Terpenes are a class of aromatic hydrocarbons found in cannabis and other plants. Terpenes in general are related to flavor and taste.

On the opposite spectrum of purchasing pure isolates and ingesting them, a whole array of edibles and beverages are on the market.

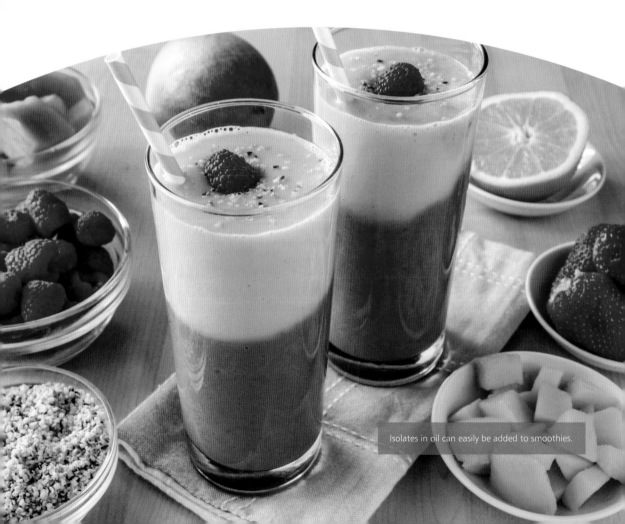

Isolates in oil can easily be added to smoothies.

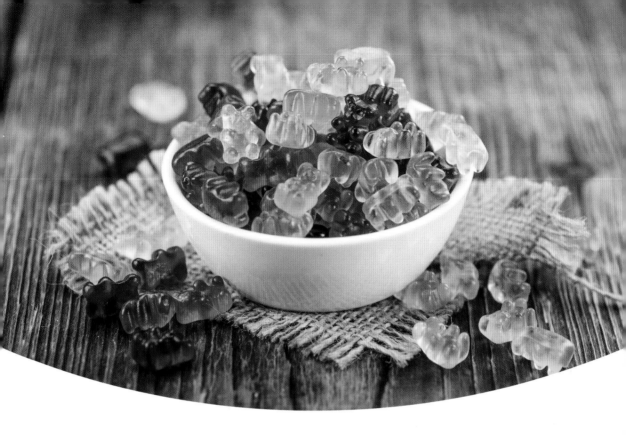

# CBD Edibles

A wide array of edible CBD products is available in stores and online. They're typically touted by companies to help with relaxation, stress relief, pain reduction, insomnia, PMS, and other health conditions. It's important to read the labels to see the amount of CDB contained in the product and other information.

For example, a bag of CBD-infused gummy bears sold online indicates on the label that each piece of candy contains a specific amount of CBD and not to eat more than two pieces every six hours. (See more on dosing on page 68.) The label also states the product is not to be sold to anyone who's under the age of 21.

Just as with the oils, tinctures, and isolates, the companies that sell these products also often indicate where the industrial hemp is grown to make the items, whether it's organic hemp, and if it's been formulated by pharmacists and tested in laboratories.

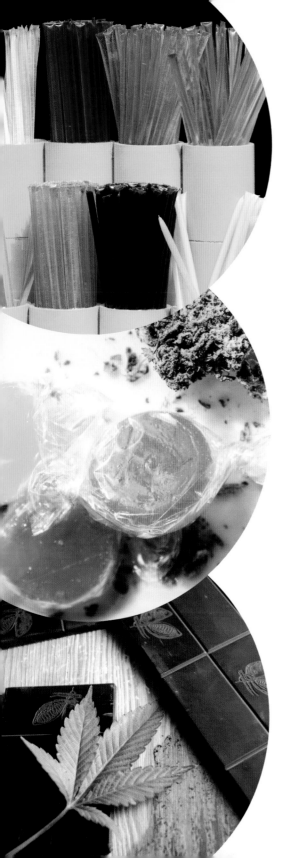

The Luce Farm in Vermont, among other businesses, makes CBD-infused honey from the hemp it grows on some of its 206 acres. The honey is sold as a sweetener for tea or coffee, or to be eaten straight from the jar. It also can be used in recipes that call for honey, as well as on cereal, toast, yogurt, and granola. Luce Farm also sells coconut oil infused with CBD. Hemp honey sticks and honey straws are also available, and can be used to dip into hot drinks or sucked on like hard candy.

Cannabinoid Creations sells a variety of CBD hard candies including blue raspberry and pomegranate lemonade. The owner founded the business after discovering that CBD oil worked better in alleviating pain from a serious injury compared with narcotics. The company also sells CBD-infused flavored syrups, suggesting a spoonful at night will help you sleep better.

Hemp CBD chocolate, of course, is very popular, and said to help with anxiety, insomnia, PMS, and depression.

You can find tins of hemp dark chocolate bark; raw black and white hemp chocolate; cocoa hemp dark chocolate bars; hemp cashew, cocoa, fruit and nut bars; chocolate hemp heart-shaped bites; dark chocolate espresso chews—and the list goes on. These CBD chocolates are often called not-pot chocolates, because they don't contain mood-altering TCH found in pot. Those who want suggested benefits from CBD oil by eating chocolates should check the label for ingredients. Some of the chocolates contain hemp seeds, but no CBD oil.

If chocolate isn't your thing, you can choose from a variety of other types of candy such as fruit-flavored CBD-infused gumdrops, breath mints, chewing gum, and CBD-infused watermelon slices.

Some companies sell bundles to try CBD in various ways. For example, one bundle contains a pain rub, a small bag of gummies, and an e liquid. The vape pen would have to be purchased separately. Another bundle might include gummies, capsules, oil, and syrup.

# CBD Beverages

Cannabinoid Creations sells hemp-infused water online as well as hemp-infused sodas in various flavors including honeydew melon, ginger ale, and grape limeade. Sprig sells wholesale CBD sodas either sweetened with sugar or flavored with stevia. Its no-sugar flavors include citrus and melon. Consumers cannot order Sprig CBD sodas online, but the drinks can be obtained at restaurants, health food stores, and other establishments in California, New York, Florida, Nevada, and Illinois.

Coca Cola is getting involved, too. It announced in 2018 that it's watching the rise of CBD beverage sales and considering whether it wants to get in the market.

You can also find a variety of CBD teas, both in the loose leaf and bag form, as well as CBD-infused coffee. One company selling the beverages states that drinking a certain amount of hemp tea daily can improve the immune system and aid in good sleep. Both the CBD-infused teas and coffees are said to improve digestion, stabilize blood sugar levels, and lower cholesterol.

Luce Farm is also experimenting with making CDB-infused beer. Don't confuse this with marijuana-infused beer, which is only legal in a few states, because it contains THC.

These CBD beverages are not inexpensive. For example, 7 tea bags infused with CBD cost $31.99 at one online store, and an 8 oz. bag of CBD-infused coffee online cost $39.99. A four-pack of 7-ounce sodas cost $28 online at one company.

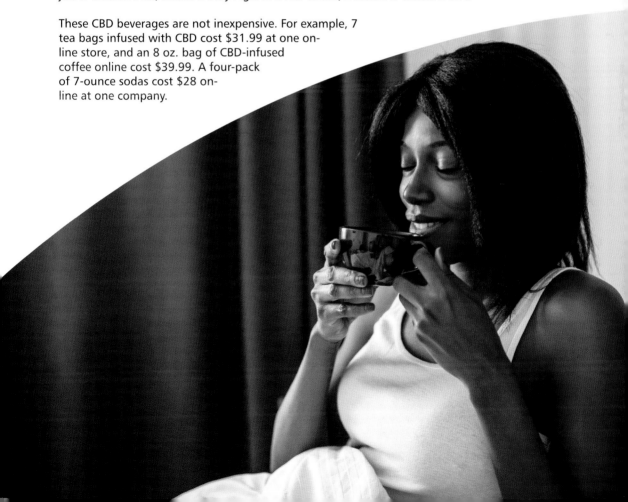

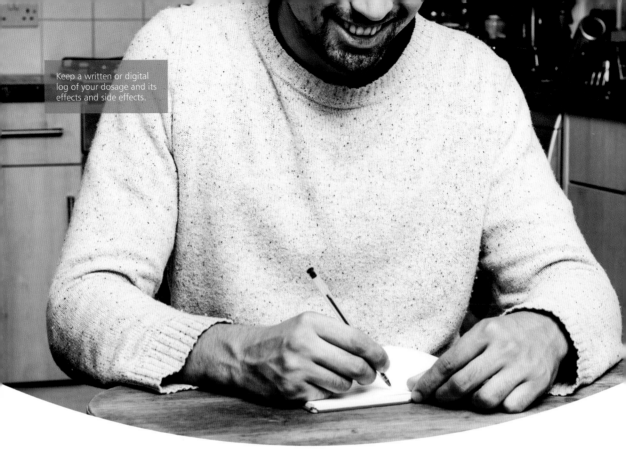
Keep a written or digital log of your dosage and its effects and side effects.

# Dosing

To get the desired effect, you'll need to consider what dosage to take—it could take up to several weeks to find the dosage that works best for you. Experts advise consulting your physician first before considering taking CBD oil to manage health issues.

When ingested, a beginning serving is from about 5 to 30 mg of CBD, but there's no official serving size because the cannabinoid is not regulated by the FDA. Taking one eyedropper per day on a label doesn't really mean a lot. In other words, you need to do your homework to determine what's best for you. That means taking into account the concentration of CBD in the product, your weight, and what condition is being treated. In addition, the right amount of CBD can change as your body changes.

Here's one way to figure out your dosage for pain using the weight method. For every 10 pounds you weigh, take 1–6 mg of CBD to start, then gradually increase until the desired effect is achieved. Someone who weighs 150 pounds, for example, would start with 15–90 mg per day, depending on the severity of the pain. It's recommended to start with small dosages and gradually increase, noting the effects on a written log.

Some experts say dosing is not that straightforward, and that using your weight as a guide might not be advised. But most agree that starting slowly, about 5 mg once or twice daily, is key. If you don't feel any effects after several days, try boosting the dosage up to about 10 mg once or twice daily. You may need to stay on that dosage for several weeks and see how it affects you before considering if you need to take more. Some experts consider more than 100 mg per day to be a high dosage. Also note that whether you take CBD on an empty stomach or after eating can have an effect. It makes sense to take the CBD the same way at the same time each day.

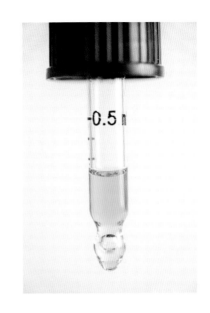

Dosages also depend on if you're using CBD oil or isolates and whether you're mixing the two, so it can be complicated. Keep a log and document what you're taking and your reactions. When dosing, you'll also want to consider what ailment you are trying to treat. It may seem counterintuitive, but CBD oil can either help you sleep, reduce anxiety, or provide you with energy depending on how much you take and when.

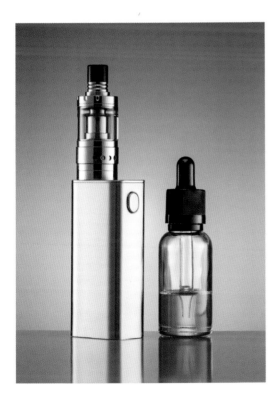

You need to be able to accurately measure your dosage—and with all the products out there, that can be difficult. But by reading the labels to see how much CBD is contained per dropper full, you can use a little math to figure it out. Labels also often will say how many milligrams are contained in the entire bottle and how many drops are in the bottle. Then you can divide to find out how much is in each drop you take.

When vaping, make sure you know how often you're refilling the tank so you know how much you're using daily.

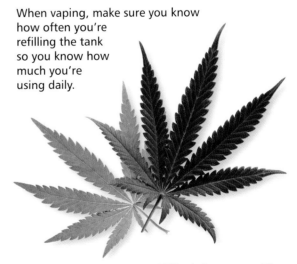

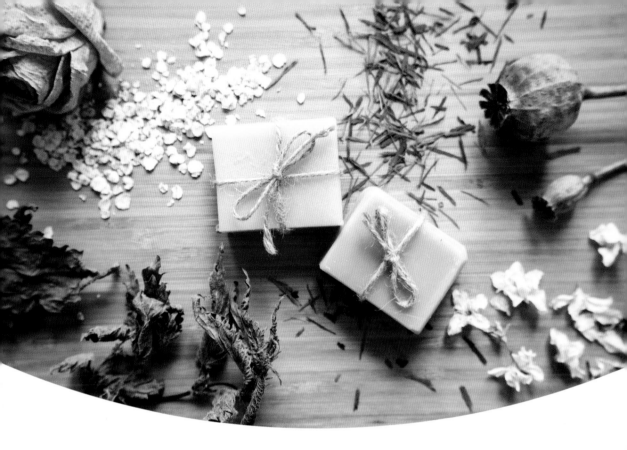

# Beauty

CBD oil isn't just for edibles—it's also infused into beauty and cleansing products. CBD oil is considered to contain antioxidants that slow age-related skin changes and heal skin conditions such as acne.

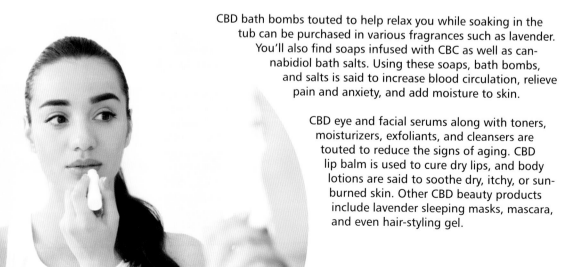

CBD bath bombs touted to help relax you while soaking in the tub can be purchased in various fragrances such as lavender. You'll also find soaps infused with CBC as well as cannabidiol bath salts. Using these soaps, bath bombs, and salts is said to increase blood circulation, relieve pain and anxiety, and add moisture to skin.

CBD eye and facial serums along with toners, moisturizers, exfoliants, and cleansers are touted to reduce the signs of aging. CBD lip balm is used to cure dry lips, and body lotions are said to soothe dry, itchy, or sunburned skin. Other CBD beauty products include lavender sleeping masks, mascara, and even hair-styling gel.

# Hemp CBD Sleep Aids

A wide variety of CBD products are specifically sold to help those with insomnia, as an alternative to taking sleeping pills. These include flavored syrups or powders that you add to beverages.

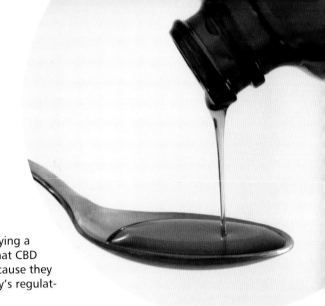

CBD products have not been clinically shown to treat insomnia and it's best to talk to your physician first about sleep problems before trying a CBD product. However, it does make sense that CBD products would help with sleep disorders, because they contain cannabinoids that work with the body's regulating system, which includes sleeping patterns.

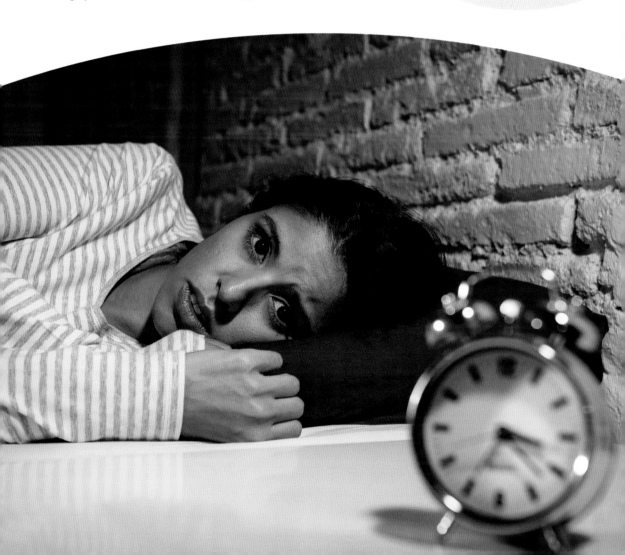

# CBD for Pets

CBD oil is said to have similar benefits for pets as it does for humans. The oil is said to help cats and dogs experiencing pain or barking or meowing excessively, as well as to help them relax them before going to the vet. Be careful with dosages and start slow, with perhaps 1 milligram per 10 pounds of body weight, increasing if needed. Consider spacing out the amount during the day in lower doses for potentially better outcomes. An Australian veterinarian has indicated he's seen CBD oil help improve a heart murmur and arthritis in a Jack Russell terrier dog. Some veterinarians recommend giving CBD oil to a dog in tincture form rather than purchasing treats infused with

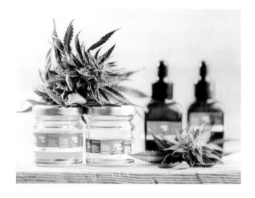

CBD. A veterinarian in Colorado has treated her feline patients with CBD oil for asthma and irritable bowel syndrome. Before administering any type of CBD to your pet, talk with your veterinarian. If your pet is taking prescribed medication, you'll need to find out from the veterinarian if CBD will change the effect of the drug.

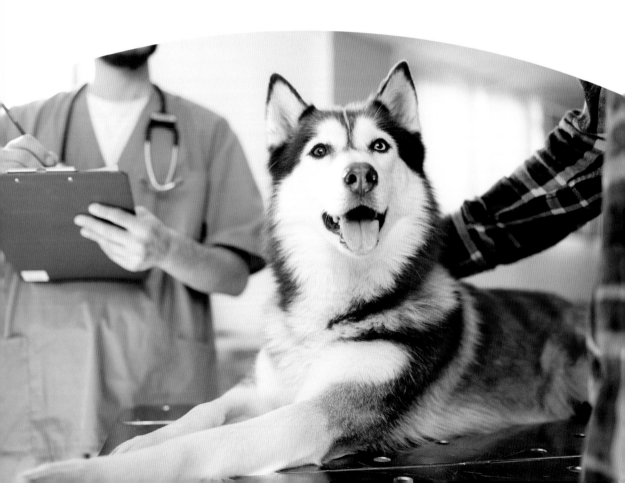

# Cooking with CBD

CBD oil as well as isolates can be used in cooking. For example, you can make chocolate chip cookies with an unflavored CBD tincture, or a carrot cake with a cinnamon-flavored CBD tincture. You might wonder why not use CBD in all the ways mentioned above instead of cooking with it. It's one way to slowly introduce CBD into your system rather than taking concentrated oils. Also, some people prefer to cook with CBD rather than take it in its many other forms. Keep in mind though that you need to be careful with the amount you use because CBD can act as sedative depending on how you use it.

You can start by sprinkling CBD isolates onto or stirring CBD oil into a smoothie, yogurt, guacamole, spaghetti sauce, soup, even chocolate chip cookie batter, as well as foods as diverse as cranberry sauce, mashed potatoes, and meatballs.

But note two important things: you need to stir the CBD very well so it is distributed evenly in the food. Also, while warming the oil can increase CBD's effectiveness, when the temperature reaches about 320 degrees Fahrenheit and higher, CBD will begin to evaporate and lose its effectiveness. In addition, it will most likely taste very bitter. Another important rule is to never put CBD oil or isolates on direct heat.

CBD also won't work effectively without fat, so choose a recipe with oil, butter, or some other fatty ingredient when cooking with it. Find out the serving size on the recipe so you know how much CBD to use. For example, if you put 50 milligrams total of CBD in a brownie recipe that makes 24 servings, each serving will have 2 milligrams of CBD in it.

Make sure to bake brownies and other CBD-infused goodies below 320 Fahrenheit. That means you might have to adjust the cooking time to compensate for lower temperature settings.

Sauces and garnishes work particularly well with CBD oil. The CB Distillery suggests using the following ingredients to make a salad dressing infused with CBD: ½ cup balsamic vinegar, ¼ cup local wildflower honey, ¼ cup extra virgin olive oil or Kalamata cold pressed olive oil, 0.25 grams CBD isolate powder, and sea salt and black pepper to taste.

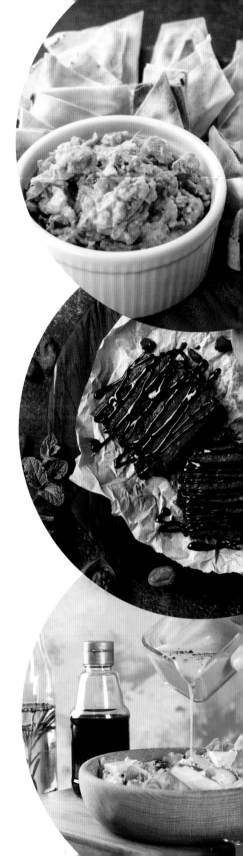

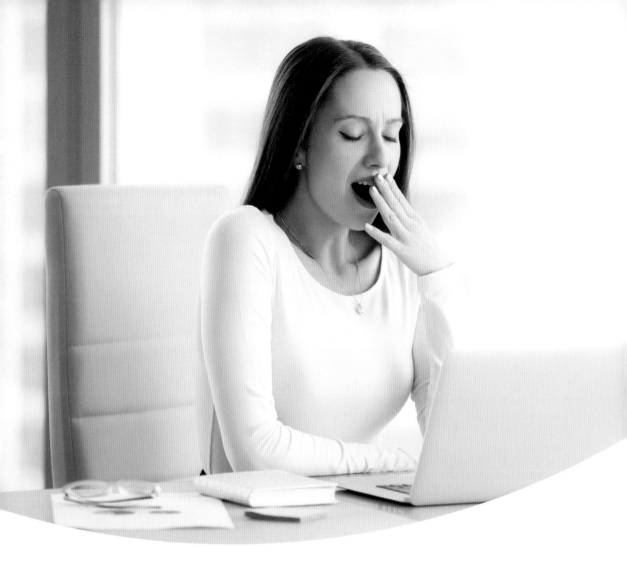

# Side Effects and Drug Interactions

CBD oil doesn't pose much of a risk to most users, but you can experience some unwanted side effects. High doses of CBD oil can slow your metabolism, meaning other drugs such as those prescribed by your doctor may not be processed as quickly. Talk with your pharmacist or physician about any potential drug interactions with CBD oil and isolates.

CBD inhibits an enzyme that helps metabolize various drugs, according to Project CBD. Some drugs said to interact with cannabidiol include steroids, antihistamines, HIV antivirals, antibiotics, antidepressants, and NSAIDs. The effects can be mild to potent depending on the dosage of CBD and drug you are taking. CBD oil can lower your blood pressure right after consuming it—and if your blood pressure is too low, you might feel light-headed. Talk to your doctor if you're taking blood pressure medication to make sure the oil won't disrupt the effects of your other drugs.

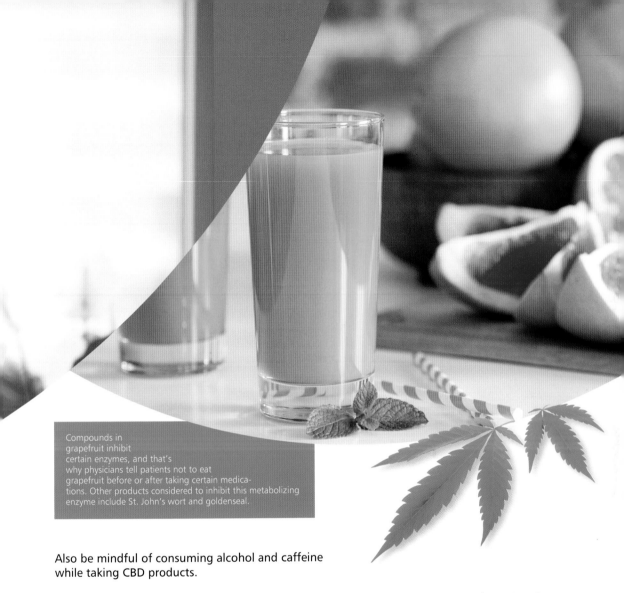

Compounds in grapefruit inhibit certain enzymes, and that's why physicians tell patients not to eat grapefruit before or after taking certain medications. Other products considered to inhibit this metabolizing enzyme include St. John's wort and goldenseal.

Also be mindful of consuming alcohol and caffeine while taking CBD products.

You can also experience dry mouth and greater thirst when using hemp CBD products. People who take CBD oil could experience diarrhea as well as increased hunger.

In addition, CBD hemp products could make you feel drowsy—which might be what you want if you're taking it to help with insomnia. But you'll need to be careful when driving or operating heavy machinery. As with any drug, seeing how it affects you first before getting behind the wheel is important. Starting with smaller doses and increasing until you get the desired effects makes sense.

As for the potential for addiction, the World Health Organization has stated that CBD does not cause humans to abuse the product or become dependent on it.

# Before You Purchase

Knowing that CBD oil products are not regulated makes it important to get the most information you can about a product before purchasing it. Ask questions of the manufacturer, read labels, and don't believe all the hype you read on line.

Here are some guidelines.

Find out how and where the industrial hemp plant used to make the product is grown. Hemp plants like others that produce cannabinoids absorb many substances from the soil in which they are growing. That means contaminants such as pollutants or metals in the soil can enter the plant. Find out if the plants are grown using pesticides, fertilizers, and other chemicals.

Every cannabinoid product out there has different amounts of CBD as well as THC. Find out by reading labels and researching the manufacturers.

Find out what kind of testing the product undergoes. For starters, it needs to be tested for outside contamination. Independent accredited labs do the best job in testing the product for safety and quality.

Read the list of ingredients. Balms, salves, edibles, and beauty products all can contain extra ingredients. For example, you might find a salve that contains apricot kernel oil, grape seed oil, arnica, vitamin E, and other products.

Read labels. Here's an example of what you might find out about a cannabinoid product by reading labels or reading about it in books or online.

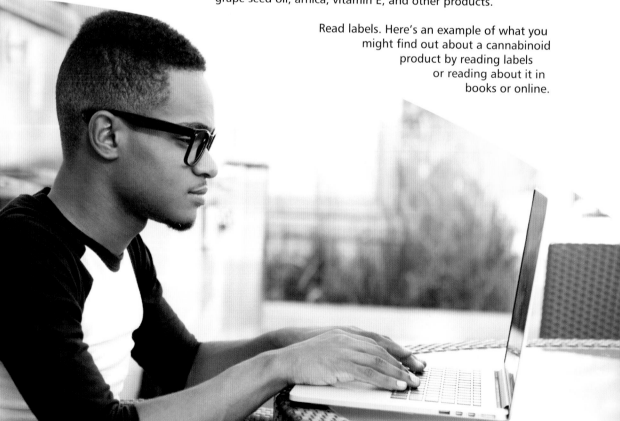

# CBD oil full spectrum peppermint spray

**CONCENTRATION:** 100 mg full-spectrum blend of CBD oil and cannabinoids

Full-spectrum means the CBD was likely extracted using carbon dioxide, and that it has not been isolated to remove any fats such as omega 3s.

**SERVING SIZE:** 1 mg CBD per two sprays

If you want to take 10 mg of CBD per day, you'll need 20 sprays.

**CARRIER:** Extra virgin olive oil

Oils, sprays and tinctures have carriers—and this one uses olive oil.

**FLAVOR:** Peppermint

Is this a natural peppermint flavor or synthesized? It would be good to find out.

**EXTRACTION PROCESS:** Supercritical CO2 Extraction

Use the information on extraction process in this book to help you understand how the oil was obtained. Supercritical CO2 extraction means the oil was extracted from the whole plant using carbon dioxide.

**LOCATION:** European grown hemp

This is industrial hemp grown out of the country. As more is grown in the U.S., depending on federal regulations, it's likely that will be a good choice because of laws that might require certain techniques or strains be used by growers.

**THIRD-PARTY LABORATORY TESTING:** This product has been third-party laboratory tested by SC Labs and verified for quality assurance through our third-party verification, Verified Life Cycle. The products are free of micro-biologics, pesticides and herbicides, residual solvents, and heavy metals.

This statement is to ensure you're receiving a high-quality product. Purchasing a product that has been tested in an independent lab is a good idea.

Another important consideration is cost—CBD oil and products made from it can be expensive. One reason is because many CBD oils are manufactured with industrial hemp from other countries, which brings up the cost. But states are starting to grow hemp again and Vermont has adopted a program in which CBD oil prices will be set throughout state-run dispensaries. That may help to keep the cost in check at least in that state.

Also remember the highest quality way of extracting the oil from the plant involves expensive equipment and trained workers, plus the best manufacturers have their products independently tested at a lab. The adage, you get what you pay for, is especially true when purchasing CBD oil. You want to get it from a reputable business that explains 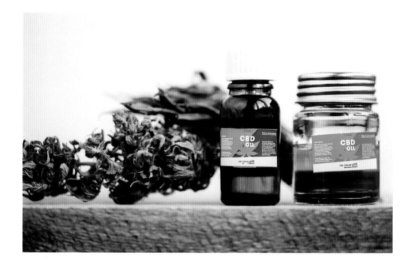 how the product is sourced and made. An online view of prices shows an average of about $30 for 300 milligrams of CBD oil. CBD imported from overseas may cost less, but it also could be of lower quality. In some online stores, you can get 1,000 milligrams of CBD isolate for the same price as 300 milligrams of CBD oil. Do your homework and read about the companies that sell oils, isolates, and edibles.

Finally, be wary of any potential black market CBD products, sold under such names as K2 and spice since the early 2000s. These products are said to be dangerous to your health.

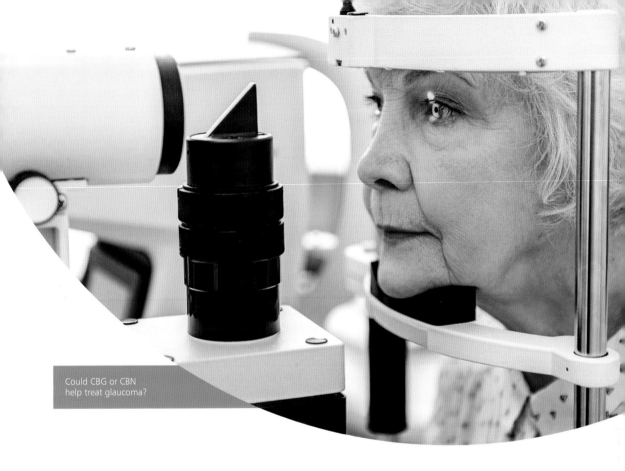

Could CBG or CBN
help treat glaucoma?

# Future Use of Other Cannabinoids

As noted in a previous section, other types of cannabinoids besides CBD and THC are found in the Cannabis plant as well as other plants. Three of these that scientists are starting to study include cannabigerol or CBG; cannabinol or CBN; and cannabichrome or CBC.

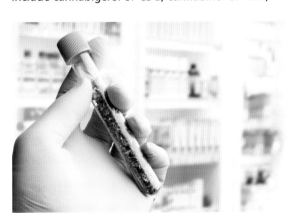

One of the scarcest cannabinoids in the cannabis plant is cannabigerol, which just like CBD, does not produce a high. Some scientists believe CBG might be able to help lower ocular pressure. High pressure in the eye can be an indicator of glaucoma. CBG also may be able to help slow muscle spasms and fight cancer cells.

CBC also is non-intoxicating and is being explored for the way it works with other cannabinoids. It could have antifungal and antibacterial properties and might be able to be used to treat the MRSA virus. Some studies suggest it also might be able to be used to treat depression and anxiety; and some even believe it could pave the way for new Alzheimer's treatments.

CBN does have some psychoactive properties, though much less than what's in THC. Some studies show that combined with other cannabinoids it can also have health benefits. When used with CBD and CBG, it may be able to treat psoriasis. CBN also may be able to reduce pain, especially when used in conjunction with CBD. CBN also may reduce inflammation and it may be able to improve sleep and even treat those with sleep disorders. Other researchers think CBN may be able to prevent glaucoma and treat epilepsy, as well as stimulate bone growth.

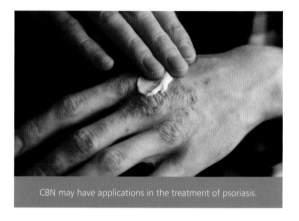
CBN may have applications in the treatment of psoriasis.

Researchers are also addressing the issue of the ratio of CBD and THC in different products, and what might work best for different ailments. For one example, in treating children with attention deficit disorder, one expert recommends using a CBD:THC ratio of 24:1. Trying to find out how that translates to which products you buy can be difficult; and a physician may be able to help.

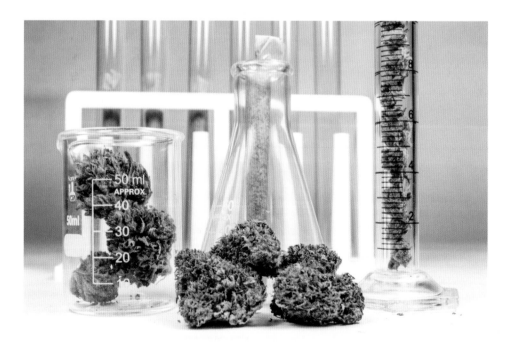

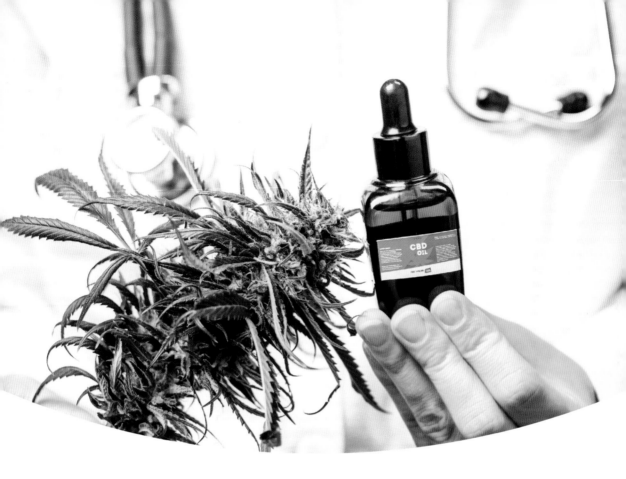

# Controversies and the Future of CBD

In September 2018, a school district in Florida told a 6-year-old girl that she could not take CBD oil when at school. Officials said the oil is a controlled substance under federal law. The girl uses the oil to control symptoms of a fatal disease, and her parents want the school to change its policy.

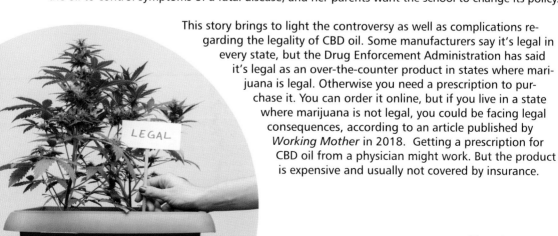

This story brings to light the controversy as well as complications regarding the legality of CBD oil. Some manufacturers say it's legal in every state, but the Drug Enforcement Administration has said it's legal as an over-the-counter product in states where marijuana is legal. Otherwise you need a prescription to purchase it. You can order it online, but if you live in a state where marijuana is not legal, you could be facing legal consequences, according to an article published by *Working Mother* in 2018. Getting a prescription for CBD oil from a physician might work. But the product is expensive and usually not covered by insurance.

Some analysts say as the CBD market grows, pharmaceutical companies will want a piece of the pie. Consider that in June 2018 the FDA approved the drug Epidiolex, a strawberry-flavored syrup that contains CBD oil, to be used to treat two rare forms of childhood epilepsy, when combined with other epilepsy drugs. It's the first prescription CBD drug approved by the FDA, and that act likely will open the door for more research on pharmaceutical drugs that can be developed using CBD to treat various diseases. It's also non-synthetic, which means it's made directly from the hemp plant.

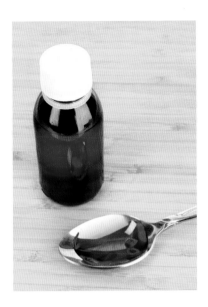

The drug, however, according to some parents whose children take it, has side effects including diarrhea, fatigue, and sleep issues. A European study published in 2017 listed diarrhea, fatigue, and changes in weight and appetite as possible side effects of CBD. Most of the research for the study published by the National Center for Biotechnical Information was conducted on those with epileptic or psychotic disorders.

Some consumers also wonder if they can just purchase CBD oil on the market and use it instead of Epidiolex, and save some money. The drug is expensive. FDA commissioner Scott Gottlieb has warned consumers not to use CBD products without proven health benefits.

In a study published in 2017, the World Health Organization's Expert Committee on Drug Dependence, however, said CBD may benefit people diagnosed with the following health issues: Alzheimer's disease, Parkinson's disease, multiple sclerosis, depression, cancer, inflammatory bowel disease, and Crohn's disease, among others. And some physicians think CBD is useful because it addresses the cause of the disease rather than merely treating the symptoms.

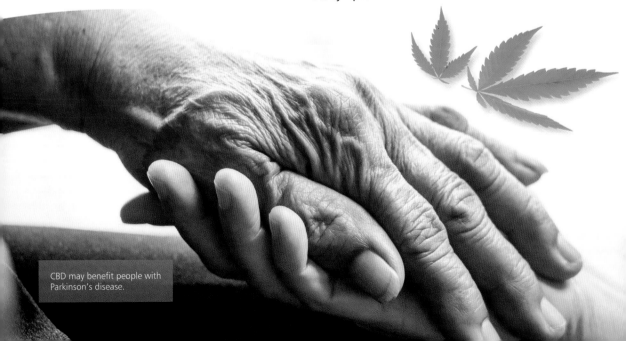

CBD may benefit people with Parkinson's disease.

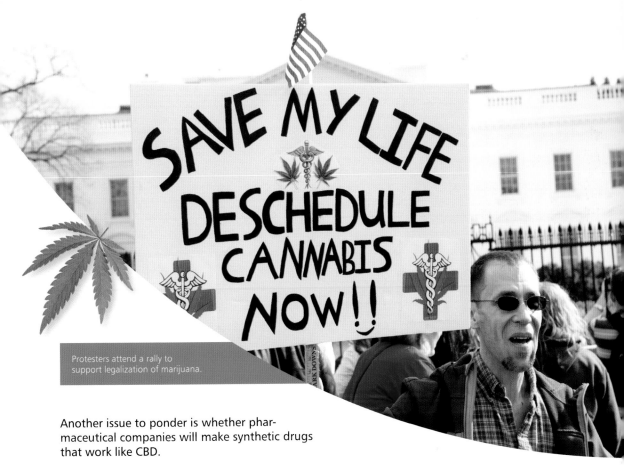

Protesters attend a rally to support legalization of marijuana.

Another issue to ponder is whether pharmaceutical companies will make synthetic drugs that work like CBD.

Already approved by the FDA is artificial THC that has been used in drugs to minimize the nausea and other side effects from chemotherapy treatment. Whether artificial cannabis can work as well as the real thing is up for debate.

The Hemp Farming Act is expected to pass sometime in 2019. If and when it does, the FDA may begin creating labeling rules and regulations for retailers who sell CBD products. Some experts think that could be a good practice because it would ensure consumers get higher quality products. Others think pharmaceutical companies will develop more artificial or synthetic forms of the cannabinoids, and wonder how that would affect sales of CBD oils on the market now.

The hope by those who promote CBD oil is that industrial hemp, from which CBD oil is made, will be legal to sell and possess without any federal repercussions in the near future. But states still have their own laws, so the complexity of the issue will continue. The bottom line, though, is that the discovery of the endocannabinoid system and research done regarding how cannabinoids play a role in this system is leading to more and more research, including the study of how combining cannabinoids might be the best way to use them for health benefits.

The next section of this book explores the various maladies touted either anecdotally or via studies that can be helped with proper dosages of CBD oil and isolates made from industrial hemp.

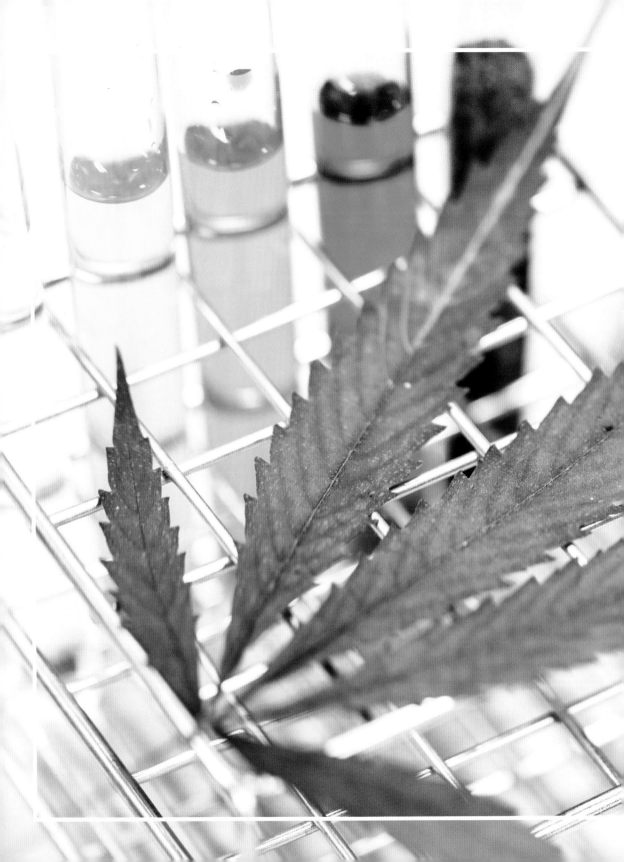

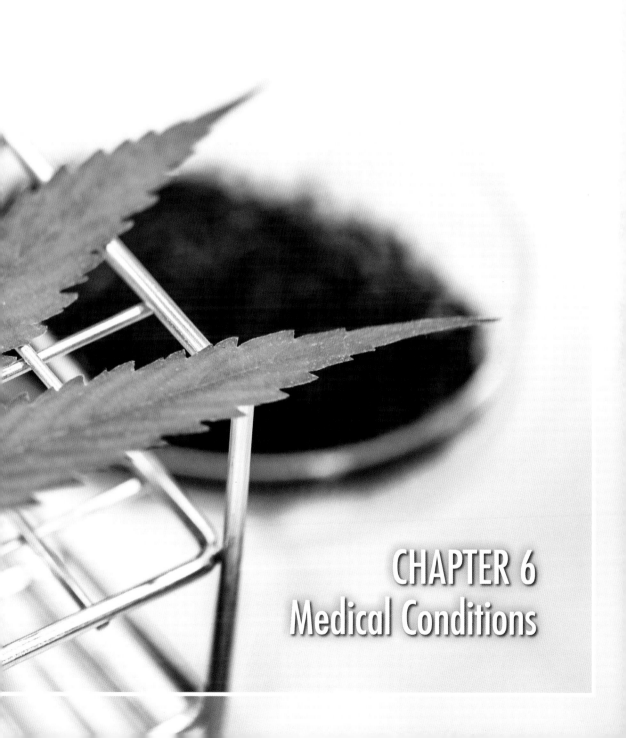

# CHAPTER 6
## Medical Conditions

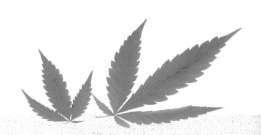

# ADHD

Up to eleven percent of children—and five percent of adults—exhibit behavior and feelings that can disrupt normal life and make it difficult to function at school, home, work, or with friends. These people are often diagnosed with one of three types of attention deficit hyperactivity disorder or ADHD.

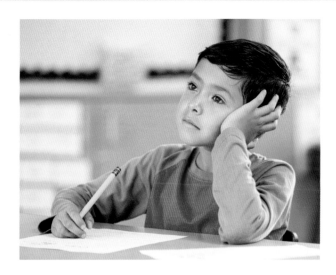

The three types include an inattentive type, a hyperactivity/impulsive type, and a combination type. As the name suggests, the inattentive type is characterized by an inability to pay attention. Those who have this type of ADHD may have a difficult time staying focused on tasks, make careless mistakes, fail to follow instructions, and can be disorganized, distracted, and forgetful. With the hyperactivity/impulsive type of ADHD, it's not uncommon to see fidgety behavior, an inability to sit still, running or climbing when it's not appropriate, and talking at inopportune times.

## ADHD Symptoms

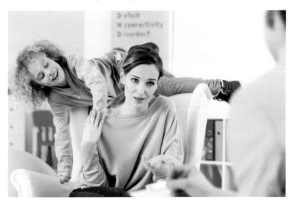

Diagnosing ADHD in children requires an evaluation with a pediatrician or psychiatrist with experience in the disorder. The physician will gather information about behavior from parents and teachers, and perform a medical evaluation to rule out any medical problems like hearing or vision disorders. Adults are often unaware that they have the disorder; they may have a history of job troubles or difficult relationships. Adults can use ADHD symptom checklists to see if they may have the condition, and talk to their doctor about a diagnosis.

# ADHD Treatment

Treatment for ADHD is usually a combination of education, psychotherapy, and medication. Surprisingly, the most common medications for the disorder are stimulants. It may seem counterproductive to use a stimulant to help someone focus or to calm fidgety behavior, but the brains of those with ADHD tend to be deficient in the neurotransmitters dopamine and norepi-

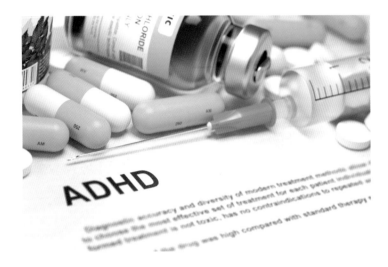

nephrine; the stimulants increase these neurotransmitters. But the medications used to treat ADHD, like Ritalin and Adderall, have been known to cause many side effects, such as nervousness, insomnia, high blood pressure, and a decrease in appetite. Long-term effects of these drugs also have not been studied.

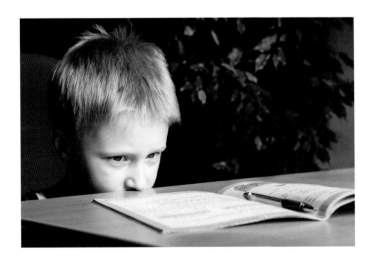

Another problem with so many young people using these drugs exists: Between three and eight percent of high school seniors have admitted to taking the drugs without a prescription, using them as a way to improve mental focus before big exams. Some teenagers have even faked ADHD symptoms to get the drugs.

# ADHD and CBD

Research into the effectiveness of CBD oil for the disorder is in its early stages. Some anecdotal evidence has shown it could work and conjectures have been made that CBD helps to regulate dopamine. A junior high school boy who suffered from ADHD and Tourette syndrome found taking CBD oil helped ease his anxiety better than a drug prescribed by his physician.

Some physicians think that in conjunction with behavioral therapy and stress-management techniques, a daily dosage of CBD oil could improve the quality of a child's life. One study showed that among adults with ADHD, thirty-four to forty-six percent have tried CBD oil.

Experts point out that no real studies have been done to show that CBD can manage symptoms of those suffering with ADHD, and any research that has been done does not show CBD oil helps manage the disorder.

A 2013 study published by *The Journal of Psychiatry* found that one third of their testing group of children with ADHD had improved after their diets were modified with fatty acid supplementation and artificial food coloring restriction, although the study also found that the children who benefited most from these modifications were children who already had restricted diets due to sensitivities.

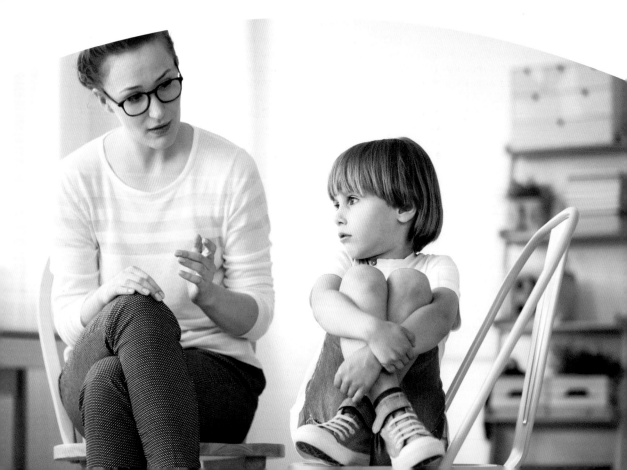

# Age-related Macular Degeneration

The leading cause of vision loss in the United States is age-related macular degeneration. It affects more than 2 million people, with experts saying the cases will grow to more than 5 million by the year 2050.

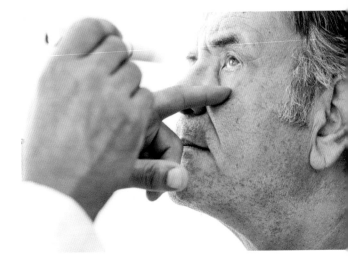

AMD, which is considered incurable, occurs when the cells of the macula in our eyes begin to deteriorate. The macula is what gives us the ability to read, drive, and recognize faces and colors. Located in the retina, the macula creates images before they're sent to the optic nerve and then to the brain.

Two types of age-related macular generation include dry and wet.

The majority have dry AMD, which happens when pieces of fat and protein collect under the retina. Wet AMD, much less common, can worsen more quickly as extra blood vessels form underneath the macula in the eye. Some experts say an overabundance of certain proteins in the eye can cause abnormal blood vessel growth, which can contribute to macular degeneration.

Experts say smoking, obesity, lack of exercise, high blood pressure, and an unhealthy diet all increase the risk of AMD. An age-related eye disease study showed that antioxidants and zinc could lower the risk for AMD. Eating leafy green vegetables and protecting your eyes from UV rays are also said to help keep the disease at bay. Annual eye exams are recommended, too.

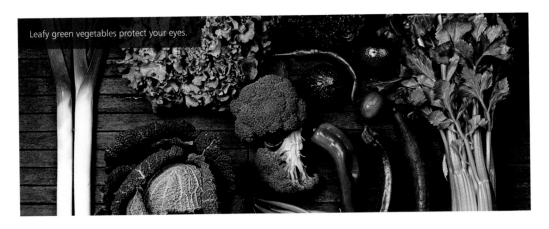

Leafy green vegetables protect your eyes.

# AMD Symptoms

In the early stages, people might have blurred vision or see wavy lines. Central vision gets lost as the disease worsens. Doctors test a patient's vision as well as look for deposits of what's called drusen beneath the retina, which is an early sign of the disease.

Patients over the age of 50 also are given what's called an Amsler grid, a pattern of straight horizontal and vertical lines. If the lines appear wavy or are missing, it could signal macular degeneration. Early detection can help slow the progression of the disease.

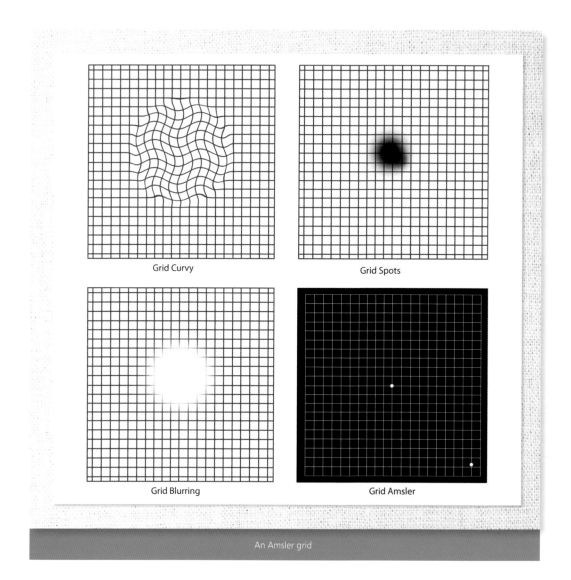

Grid Curvy

Grid Spots

Grid Blurring

Grid Amsler

An Amsler grid

# AMD Treatment

Medications that stop new blood vessels from forming can be injected into a patient's eye. The medication may help some people regain vision lost from the disease, but it can trigger side effects such as pain, infections, swelling, and other vision problems.

Another treatment is laser therapy used to destroy the abnormal blood vessels, and a third is photodynamic laser therapy, which uses a light-sensitive drug to get rid of abnormal blood vessels.

# AMD and CBD

A business owner in New Mexico started using CBD oil to help with a disease she contracted from a tick. While taking CBD oil, the woman, who had suffered from macular degeneration, noticed the symptoms from that disease seemed to be lessening. When she saw her eye doctor, one of her eyes had improved—and the doctor did not know she was taking CBD.

As macular degeneration progresses, it affects central vision.

Some researchers say cannabinoids have been shown to slow the growth of certain compounds in the eye that contribute to MD. They also say that CBD oil can serve as an anti-inflammatory, which can help those with MD.

A 2002 Finnish study showed that cannabinoid receptors are found in the eye; that could mean the receptors would react to the ingestion of CBD oil. CBD is also considered an anti-inflammatory for the eye and is said to inhibit the growth of new blood vessels, which contribute to the disease.

Clinical studies on how CBD oil affects those with AMD are lacking, and the use of CBD oil to ease symptoms needs much more research.

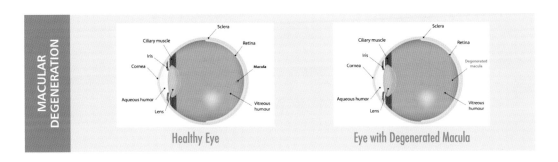

MACULAR DEGENERATION

Healthy Eye

Eye with Degenerated Macula

# Alzheimer's Disease

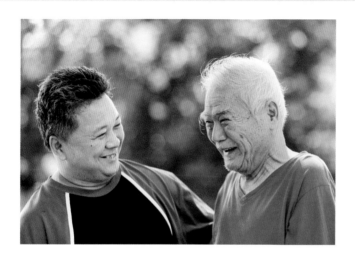

The term Alzheimer's disease often makes us think of the elderly, but this progressive disease is not a normal part of aging. In fact, this irreversible brain disorder—which destroys memory, cognition, and even the ability to perform simple everyday tasks—does not even exclusively affect older people: About 200,000 Americans under the age of sixty-five are afflicted with Alzheimer's. The youngest person to ever be diagnosed was only twenty-seven years old.

## Alzheimer's Symptoms

The classic first symptoms are memory lapses, such as misplacing objects, struggling to remember the correct word, or forgetting names; the most common symptom is failing to retain newly learned information, because the disease first attacks the part of the brain responsible for learning. Unfortunately, Alzheimer's disease doesn't stop there. The disease marches through the brain, leading to increasingly severe symptoms, including disorientation, mood changes, serious memory loss, confusion about time or place, and an inability to recognize friends, family, or caregivers. Eventually, Alzheimer's patients reach a point where they are unable to care for themselves. They can have difficulty communicating, and may lose the ability to walk, sit up, or swallow, making them especially susceptible to infections like pneumonia.

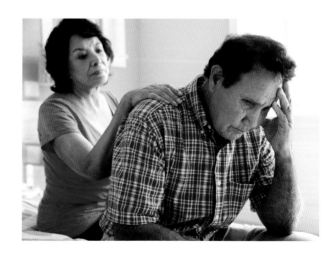

# The Progression of the Disease

Alzheimer's atrophies various regions of the brain. The loss of neurons and synapses in the cerebral cortex and other subcortical regions are the prime causes of the degradation of the temporal and parietal lobe.

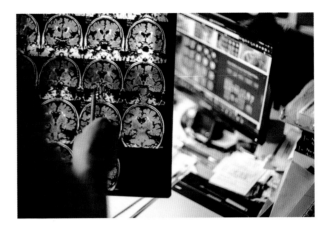

Diagnosing Alzheimer's can be very difficult, but it is often successfully diagnosed after the cognitive impairments of the disease begin to compromise the daily routine of those who suffer from it. Alzheimer's significantly affects the lives of those who suffer from it, and the lifespans of those who are diagnosed are greatly reduced. After diagnosis, the lifespan of those who are suffering from the disease is three to ten years. Less than three percent of people living with Alzheimer's live longer than fourteen years after diagnosis.

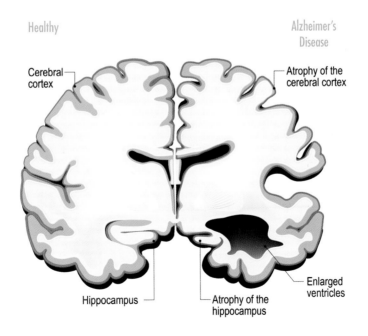

Healthy

Alzheimer's Disease

Cerebral cortex

Atrophy of the cerebral cortex

Hippocampus

Atrophy of the hippocampus

Enlarged ventricles

# Risks and Preventative Measures

While the biggest risk factors for Alzheimer's—age and a family history of the disease—can't be changed, researchers are discovering that there may be ways to prevent it. Living a healthy lifestyle is key. Eating well, exercising, and avoiding tobacco and alcohol are a good start. Studies have linked heart health to brain health, so staying on top of heart issues like high blood pressure and high cholesterol is vital.

A number of medical and lifestyle options can be taken to prevent Alzheimer's disease. Although there is no definitive evidence to support these claims, lowering your exposure to cardiovascular risk factors like high cholesterol, smoking, diabetes, and hypertension could help lower your risk of developing Alzheimer's disease. Lifestyle changes can also have a tremendous effect in preventing the onset of Alzheimer's. Mentally and physically challenging activities like reading, doing puzzles, playing games, playing musical instruments, socializing, and exercising have all been shown to lower the likelihood of developing Alzheimer's and reducing the severity of the disease's symptoms. Healthy diets, including Japanese and Mediterranean diets, can also reduce your risk of developing the disease.

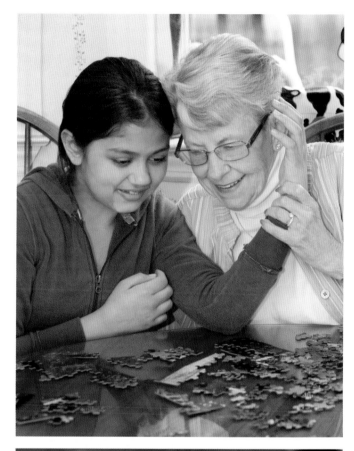

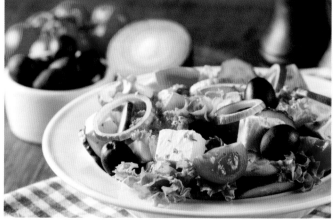

# Alzheimer's Treatment

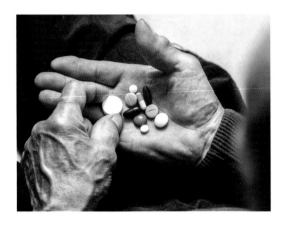

So far, Alzheimer's has no cure, and there is no way to stop the eventual progression of the disease. But treatments are available to slow it down and to abate symptoms. Medications may be prescribed that prevent the breakdown of chemicals in the brain responsible for learning and memory. These can delay the loss of independence suffered by those with Alzheimer's, prolonging their quality of life. Other medications may also be given to relieve some of the symptoms that come along with the disease: Antidepressants can lift mood and decrease irritability; antianxiety medications can ease anxiety and restlessness; and antipsychotic medications can help with aggression, hostility, or hallucinations. Some patients also add supplements like coenzyme Q10, ginkgo biloba, coral calcium, or coconut oil to their diets, although research of these is limited and there is little evidence to support their effects on Alzheimer's.

# Alzheimer's and CBD

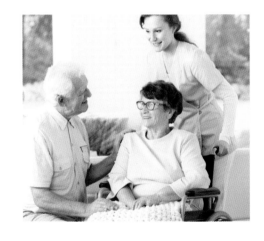

According to some studies, CBD oil has the potential to be included in a new drug regimen that might slow the progress of Alzheimer's disease. Other studies have shown CBD may be able to prevent plaque formation, which has been linked to the disease. In addition, another study done with mice showed by using CBD, the animal's memory was improved.

Alzheimer's is considered a neurodegenerative disease and contracting the disease may be related to inflammation of the body's neural tissues. CBD oil could potentially be used as an anti-inflammatory with Alzheimer's patients, which could slow the disease's progression.

Some studies are being done to determine if CBD or other cannabinoids can alleviate certain symptoms of Alzheimer's. One study unfortunately found no link between using CBD and improving certain behaviors in patients with dementia, a disease closely related to Alzheimer's.

# Amyotrophic Lateral Sclerosis (ALS)

Amyotrophic lateral sclerosis or ALS, is an incurable, progressive disease that destroys nerve cells, which leads to disability, and eventually death. An estimated 20,000 to 30,000 Americans are living with the disease.

ALS is also known as Lou Gehrig's disease, referring to the famous baseball player who developed the disease.

Physicians do not know the causes of ALS, but about five to ten percent of the people with the disease inherit it. Researchers are studying potential causes such as gene mutation, a faulty immune system, and an imbalance in the amount of glutamate in the brain.

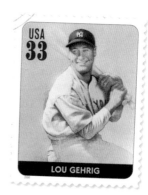

USA 33
LOU GEHRIG

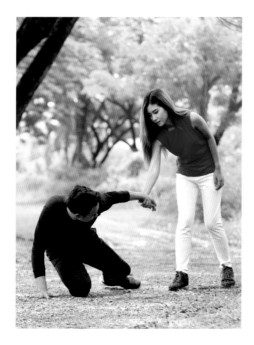

Some of the first symptoms of ALS include a weak limb, twitching muscles, slurred speech, trouble swallowing, and tripping. As the disease progresses, the patient loses the ability to move, speak, eat, and breathe.

ALS is typically diagnosed when someone is between forty and sixty years old. Risk factors include smoking, exposure to environmental toxins, and also serving in the military. Researchers conjecture that those in the military may be exposed to infections, traumatic injuries, and other situations that trigger the disease.

It's difficult to diagnose ALS because its symptom mimic other diseases; but various tests and studies can signal that a person has Lou Gehrig's disease. These include an electromyogram in which the electrical activity of muscles is studied, blood and urine tests, and magnetic resonance imaging.

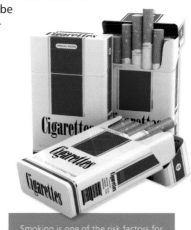

Smoking is one of the risk factors for ALS, along with other diseases.

# Treatment

Treatments can slow the disease's progression and relieve some symptoms, but they can't reverse damage done to the body. Often, several healthcare professionals work together to select treatments that work best for individual patients to live a better quality of life.

The FDA has approved two medications to treat ALS. One of them, taken in pill form, is said to slow the disease's progression, but it can cause dizziness and changes in the functioning of the liver and the gastrointestinal tract. Another, given with infusions daily for roughly ten days, has been shown to slow the decline in certain symptoms. Side effects with this drug may include bruising, swelling, and shortness of breath, as well as allergic reactions.

AMYOTROPHIC LATERAL SCLEROSIS (ALS)

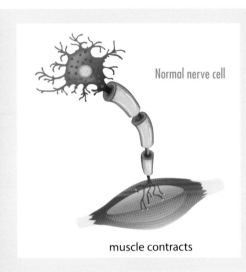

Normal nerve cell

muscle contracts

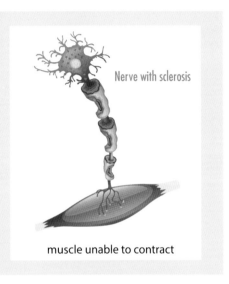

Nerve with sclerosis

muscle unable to contract

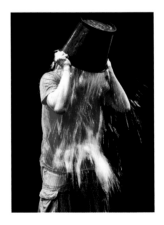

Other medications may be able to help with symptoms such as muscle cramps, fatigue, pain, depression, and uncontrolled laughing and crying.

ALS patients also receive physical, speech, and occupational therapy, as well as a ventilation apparatus to help them breathe.

Research is ongoing to find medications and treatments that can help ALS patients. In 2015, the ice-bucket challenge was launched on Facebook to raise awareness of ALS—people had buckets of ice water thrown on them, and raised more than 100 million dollars to go toward research on the disease.

# ALS and CBD

Some ALS patients have found that CBD reduces muscle spasms, and researcher say CBD may be able to help cells live longer, which could slow the disease's progression. One study also suggests some form of cannabis might be able to manage ALS symptoms such as sleep problems, muscle issues, and lack of appetite.

Researchers also are considering how other cannabinoids besides CBD might be able to help ALS patients. For example, CBD or canna-bichromene may promote brain growth. CBC, like CBD, comes from the cannabis plant, and researchers are looking at how dif-ferent cannabinoids may work together to help with various diseases and conditions.

Some anecdotal evidence shows that marijuana may help patients with ALS, which has prompted researchers to call for studies on whether the non-hallucinogenic CBD can help as well.

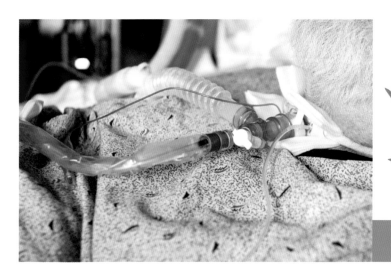

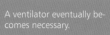

A ventilator eventually be-comes necessary.

# Arthritis

Arthritis encompasses more than one hundred types of afflictions that can affect people of all ages. More than 50 million adults and 300,000 children have some type of the disease, which is the leading cause of disability in the United States. Symptoms can include swelling, pain, and stiffness in one or more joints, as well as a decreased range of motion. Although the symptoms may come and go at first, over time, pain from arthritis can become chronic, making performing normal everyday tasks—like opening jars, climbing stairs, or even walking—difficult and uncomfortable.

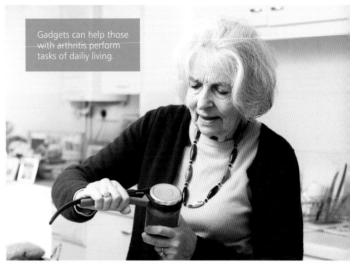

Gadgets can help those with arthritis perform tasks of dailiy living.

According to the Centers for Disease Control and Prevention, women are more likely to suffer from arthritis than men. Old age also plays a role in the probability of being diagnosed with the disease.

# Osteoarthritis

The most common type of arthritis is osteoarthritis. In this degenerative disease, the cartilage between bones wears away until bone rubs on bone. Popular treatments include over-the-counter pain relievers, as well as using hot and cold compresses, and engaging in regular exercise to strengthen the muscles surrounding the joint.

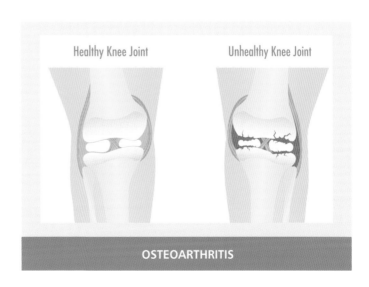

Healthy Knee Joint    Unhealthy Knee Joint

**OSTEOARTHRITIS**

# Inflammatory Arthritis

Inflammatory arthritis occurs when the immune system goes awry and begins attacking joints, as well as internal organs, eyes, and other body parts. Types include rheumatoid arthritis and psoriatic arthritis, and it can be treated with disease-modifying anti-rheumatic drugs.

Early signs and symptoms of rheumatoid arthritis are similar to those of other diseases, and no single blood test can completely confirm the presence of the disease. Physicians look for swelling, redness, and warmth in the joins and also check muscle strength and reflexes. People with rheumatoid arthritis often have what are called high sed rates, which can show there's inflammation in the body. Imaging tests also are used to determine the severity of the disease.

The goal with inflammatory arthritis is to catch it early and achieve remission in order to prevent permanent joint damage. Unfortunately, some of the drugs used can have side effects such as the risk of heart attack or stroke.

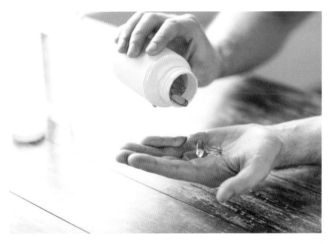

Some studies show that fish oil supplements may reduce symptoms of rheumatoid arthritis. Tai chi is also considered a potential therapy.

In extreme cases, surgery may be done to fuse or repair joints or replace tendons.

Other types of arthritis include infectious arthritis, which occurs when a bacteria, virus, or fungus causes joint inflammation, and metabolic arthritis—also called gout—which is caused by a buildup of uric acid in the body.

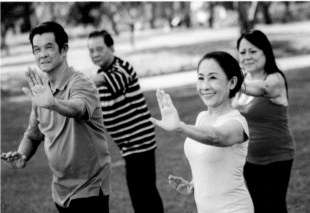

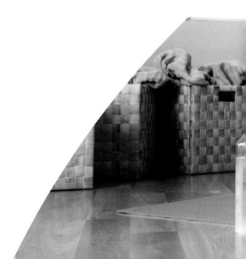

# Arthritis and CBD

Depending on the type of arthritis a patient has, CBD has been found, at least anecdotally, to counteract the pain. One patient with severe arthritis in her knee began using a CBD ointment twice a day and found her pain to be much relieved. She also said she used a CBD vaping pen. A study on treating arthritic pain in animals showed a topical treatment of CBD could reduce inflammation and pain. Another study showed patients with rheumatoid arthritis noticed less pain and inflammation after using CBD for about five weeks.

Experts recommend a dosage of about 3 to 30 mg of oral CBD oil for about 25 days to ease arthritic symptoms. But arthritis sufferers should keep in mind that not much scientific evidence exists to prove CBD effectively treats arthritis in humans, and speaking with a physician before taking CBD oil is warranted.

Researchers think CBD decreases inflammation by blocking cytokines in the body, which are triggered either by an infection or an immune system that has gone haywire.

CBD also is said to have fewer and less severe side effects compared with some of the drugs administered to treat arthritis.

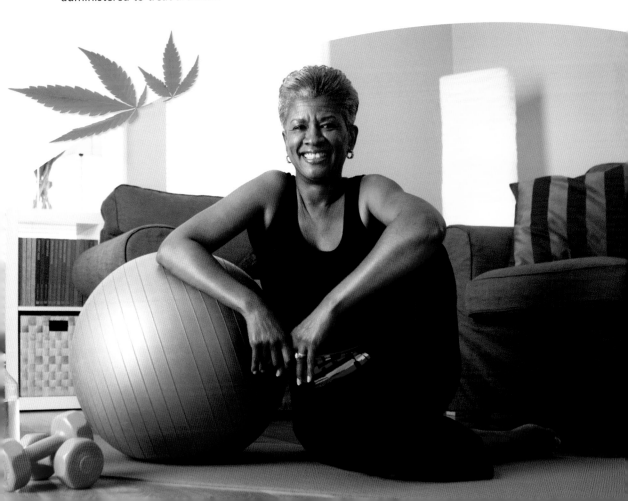

# Autism

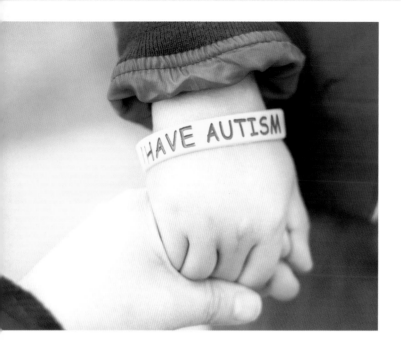

Worldwide, about one percent of children are affected with autism spectrum disorder. Autism disproportionately affects children in developed countries, with about one in fifty-nine children in the United States diagnosed with the disorder.

This disorder encompasses four different diagnoses: autistic disorder, childhood disintegrative disorder, pervasive developmental disorder-not otherwise specified, and Asperger syndrome. All of these can cause varying degrees of communication difficulties, challenges with social skills, hypersensitivities to sound or light, and repetitive behaviors.

## Symptoms of Autism

For some, the disorder can be mild, resulting in an impaired ability to read social cues, difficulty making friends, and discomfort with eye contact. Many of these children grow up to have fulfilling lives, albeit with challenges. For others, autism is much more severe. For these children, symptoms can turn harmful or violent, and include repetitive head-banging, uncontrollable tantrums and rages, insomnia, and often an inability to speak. About one third of children with autism remain nonverbal throughout their lives.

Children with autism are also prone to other medical or mental health conditions, such as ADHD, anxiety disorders, gastrointestinal disorders, seizures, and phobias. Autism has no cure, so most treatments focus on these individual symptoms. Antianxiety or antipsychotic medications may be given, as well as ADHD drugs like Ritalin. For many children, these drugs only have an effect for a few hours; after that, symptoms can become even more extreme.

Treating autism can be difficult and complicated, but so too can be diagnosing it. The disorder cannot be diagnosed with a blood test. Doctors make diagnoses by observing a child's behavior and development.

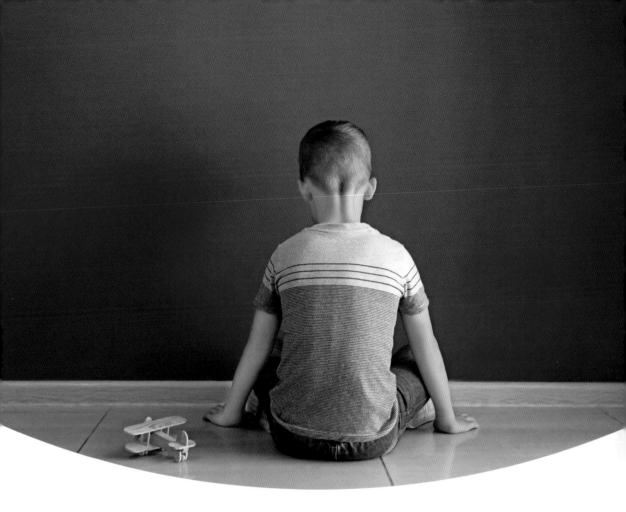

# Causes of Autism

The causes of autism are still disputed, but strong evidence exists that genetic factors play a role in diagnosis. The common worry that vaccinating children has a role in causing autism is largely disproven. Parents usually begin to notice signs of autism around the same time a child would begin to get vaccinated, causing a false correlation in the minds of parents.

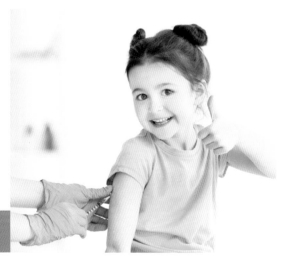

Parents can vaccinate their children without worries of autism.

# CBD Oil and Autism

Israeli researchers are conducting a study with preliminary results showing that 80 percent of children who were treated with high concentrations of CBD for at least seven months had improved. The study is based on reports from parents during and after the treatment. What they found so far was that half the children's communication improved, and more than three-quarters had fewer behavior problems. In addition, nearly half had less anxiety.

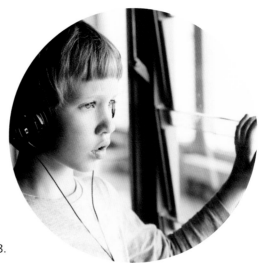

The study involves 120 patients with mild to severe autism with ages between 5 and 29 years old. The study was to continue through the end of 2018.

The president of the Autism Society of America has said that anecdotal evidence from parents shows that using CBD has helped their autistic children. But more rigorous scientific research is still needed, he said.

Studies were set to begin in spring of 2018 in New York to determine if children diagnosed with moderate to severe autism can gain health benefits from CBD. Half of the children were to be given a placebo, the other CBD. The researchers and the children were not to be told which one was received. The tests were scheduled to be done at Montefiore Medical Center and NYU Langone on patients ages 5 to 18 who were diagnosed with severe autism.

Also in 2018, a nonprofit foundation gave nearly $5 million toward research to the UC San Diego School of Medicine to conduct CBD trials on autistic children. The study will research whether treating children with autism with CBD is safe and effective.

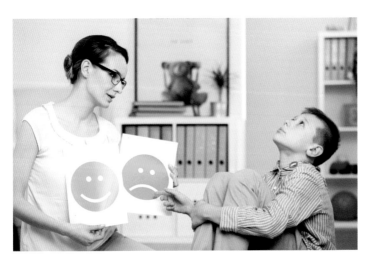

# Cancer

Few words sound as scary as cancer—hearing the diagnosis can be extremely frightening and overwhelming. For a disease that causes so much upheaval in people's lives, cancer is a surprisingly simple process: It occurs when cells in the body begin to grow out of control, crowding out normal cells and interrupting the usual functions of the body. Cancer cells can begin growing anywhere in the body, and then spread—or metastasize—to other areas.

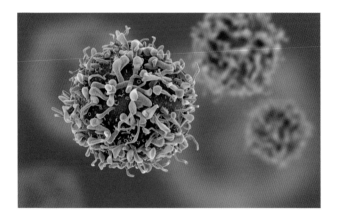

In the United States, cancer is second only to heart disease in common causes of death. Over the last forty years, approximately $90 billion has been spent on cancer research and treatment as scientists search for cures and ways to improve quality of life. And the good news is, deaths from cancer have been declining steadily for decades, falling twenty-six percent since 1991. Still, it was estimated that about 1.7 million Americans will be diagnosed with the disease in 2018, and approximately 600,000 will lose the battle.

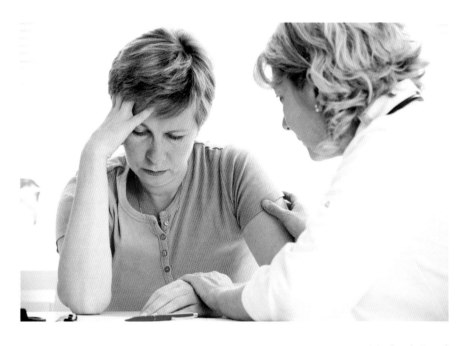

# Traditional Treatments for Cancer

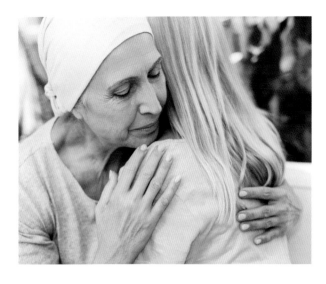

Such an insidious disease often requires aggressive treatment. Surgery can be used to remove as much cancer as possible, but often patients require chemotherapy or radiation treatments—or both. Chemotherapy is a drug therapy that aims to kill cancer cells and prevent them from multiplying. Unfortunately, the treatment can inadvertently target healthy cells as well, leading to extreme side effects like nausea and vomiting, hair loss, fatigue, a loss of appetite, and depression. Radiation therapy, which targets cancer cells with high doses of radiation, can also cause similar unpleasant side effects.

The side effects of cancer treatment can be so bad that patients are unable to live normal lives. Some patients have described feeling nauseated all day, or feeling worse than with any bout of flu they've ever had. Weight loss is common, as it can be difficult to keep food down or to even have an appetite.

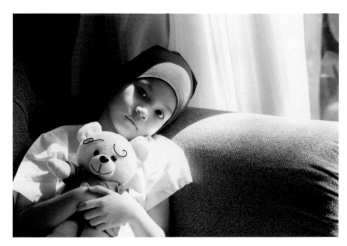

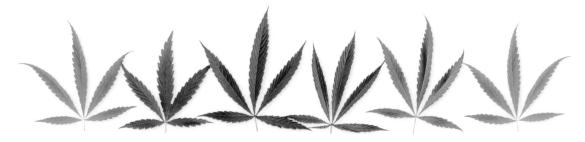

# Cancer Prevention, Treatment, Treatment of Side Effects, and CBD

Some researchers believe taking CBD oil can act as a preventative measure against cancer. One study showed, for example, that animals treated with CBD were much less likely to develop colon cancer, after being induced with the disease in a laboratory, compared with those who did not receive CBD. A British researcher said CBD might also prove to be effective in preventing colon cancer.

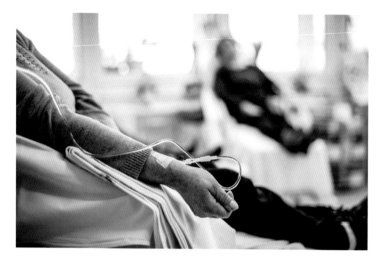

Some studies have shown that CBD could shrink tumors and halt the growth of new cancer cells. One study showed CBD might prevent cancer caused by smoking tobacco. Tests are being done on best ratios of CBD and THC to produce a drug that could slow the progress of the disease. That means that using CBD isolates, which contain no THC, might not work.

Anecdotal evidence, of course, exists, that CBD could shrink tumors, since cancer patients often are willing to try many different treatments. For example, a 39-year-old woman with brain cancer was treated with radiation and told the treatment didn't work. She began taking high doses of CBD oil, which had a ratio of 120 mg CBD to 80 mg THC. She also exercised every day and ate a specific diet. Within a year, her tumor had shrunk considerably. The woman believes a low-THC, high CBD concentrate made from the cannabis plant is what saved her.

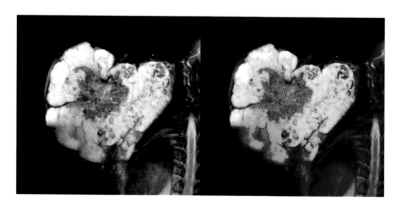

One patient diagnosed with terminal lung cancer took CBD oil for seven months and was cancer free at that point, though not much is known about how she fared after that.

One study showed that CBD inhibited tumor growth related to breast cancer, and that it might be able to be used to stop the growth of highly aggressive breast cancers. Another study showed CBD might be able to kill colon and prostate cancer cells related to the way certain enzymes work in the body.

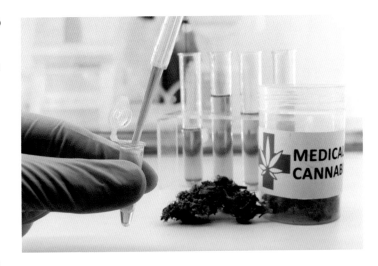

Tackling leukemia as well as skin cancers also might be able to be done with CBD. Skin cancer is one of the most common forms of cancer and every year, 3.5 million Americans are diagnosed with the disease. Some anecdotal evidence suggest topical application of CBD could help skin cancer patients, but others warn against using it.

The National Cancer Institute has said that using CBD can reduce nausea that happens after chemotherapy treatments, and patients with neuropathic pain found they could lessen their pain using an oil containing both CBD and THC. CBD oil may also be able to help patients from losing weight and restore their appetites while undergoing treatment.

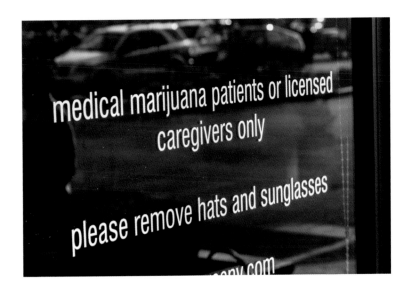

It's important to note that researchers are just beginning to study the different elements contained in CBD as well as the ratio between CBD and THC that might be the most effective in treating cancer. Where medical marijuana is legal, some patients might be able to obtain CBD that contains a higher percentage of THC than what's found in over-the-counter and online CBD oils.

# Concussions and Traumatic Brain Injuries

About one million people in the United States are treated in emergency rooms each year for traumatic brain injuries, resulting from traffic accidents, sports-related concussions, military injuries, and strokes.

People who have had repeated injuries may be more susceptible to having chronic traumatic encephalopathy, called CTE. This degenerative brain disease typically affects athletes, veterans, and others such as victims of domestic violence.

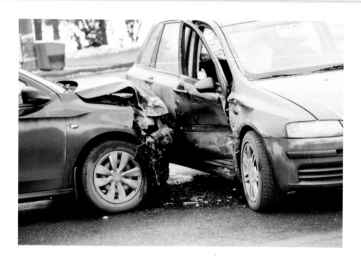

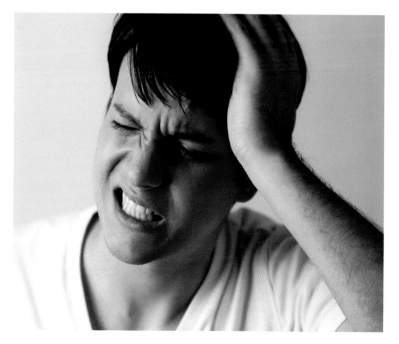

Symptoms typically begin when people are in their late twenties or early thirties. Some of these symptoms include aggression, paranoia, and depression, followed later by memory loss, impaired judgment, and even dementia.

Researchers first described CTE in the late 1920s based on symptoms of a group of boxers. In 2005, the first case of CTE in an American football player was published.

Not everyone with repetitive hits to the head will get CTE; and if someone has only had one concussion, it's highly unlikely that person will develop the disease.

In addition, some researchers are saying that CTE is related to genetics, medical problems, drug abuse, and other issues unrelated to concussions. That makes it difficult for parents to know what to do when it comes to their children participating in athletic sports such as football.

For a long time, CTE could only be diagnosed by analyzing brain tissue after a person dies. But researchers showed a brain scan of a former National Football League player had what they called a buildup of tau proteins around damaged brain areas. The condition was formally confirmed after he died due to complications from ALS.

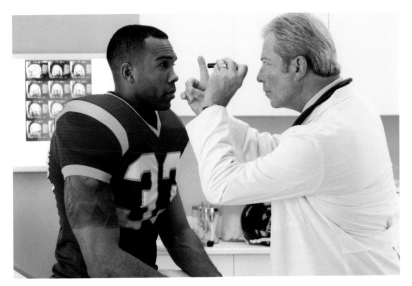

No cure is available for those with symptoms of CTE. Patients are treated for their symptoms instead. Treatments include medications, massage, acupuncture, working with a therapist on mood changes, working with an expert to improve memory, and other techniques.

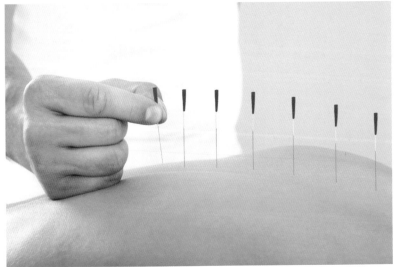

# CTE and CBD

Some preliminary studies on animals have shown that CBD might be able to help recovery after a brain injury as well as reduce headaches and anxiety associated with traumatic brain injury and concussions.

No clinical trials have proven CBD can help those with traumatic brain injuries, but some anecdotes are revealing that the potential could be there.

One physician who treats chronic brain injuries in athletes, veterans, and those involved in accidents gives them CBD along with fatty acids, which are said to promote brain health.

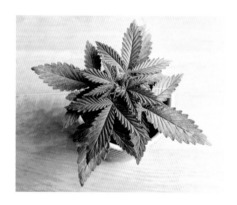

One of his patients who suffered a brain injury after a car crash tried various therapies, but depression and anxiety continued to plague him. He began taking CBD and since has stopped taking anti-depression medication and returned to his job as a performer.

Former American football player Kyle Turley believes CBD products have helped him with neurological problems associated with brain injuries. In fact, he founded a company that makes CBD products for brain health. It's called Neuro XPF and it's touted to be free of THC, which means athletes who take the product will not test positive for marijuana on drug tests.

Other NFL players including Jim McMahon have voiced their opinions on how CBD could help those with repeated brain injuries. Another angle to this controversial issue is that if CBD can alleviate pain associated with the injuries, perhaps the patients would not be taking opioids for pain, which can become addictive.

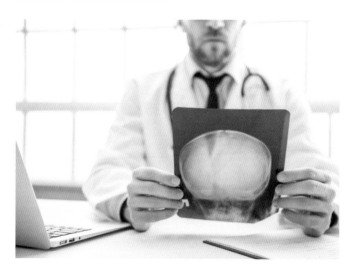

The University of Miami has received a grant for a five-year study to see if a pill with CBD can treat concussion injuries. The study was to begin sometime after 2016. Researchers are thinking combining drugs may help reduce brain inflammation on those who suffer from concussion. Much more research is needed to find out if concussions are related to CTE, and what new medications might be able to help people who suffer from symptoms of repeated traumatic brain injuries.

# Depression and Anxiety

We all feel sad or stressed out now and then; the struggles of life make sure of that. But for some individuals, those moods begin to feel overwhelming and last for weeks or months at a time, preventing them from living life to the fullest.

## Depression

Depression is characterized by several symptoms, including a sad mood, lack of energy, feelings of worthlessness, lack of focus, and sleeping disorders. People who suffer with the condition can also be irritable, eat too much or not enough, feel anxious, or even have physical symptoms like headaches, joint pain, or digestive trouble. Depression can make other physical issues—especially chronic pain—feel even worse. People who are severely depressed may often spend days in bed, too depressed to get out and approach life.

In addition, those with severe depression may contemplate suicide. In fact, suicide is one of the top causes of death in the U.S. Almost 45,000 Americans died of suicide in 2016, according to the Centers for Disease Control and Prevention, and the rates are rising.

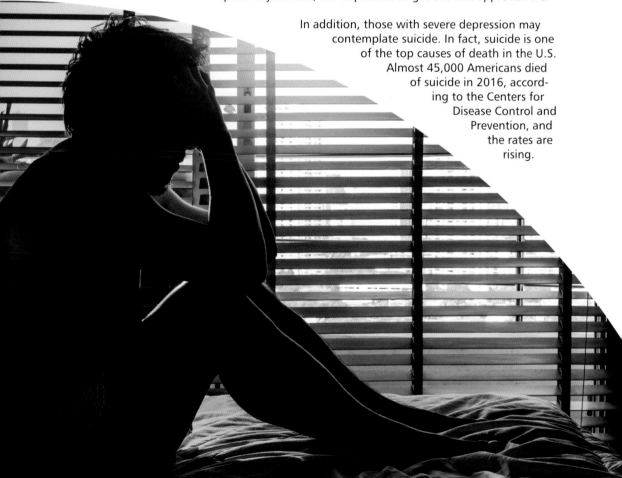

Depression can affect anyone, although women are twice as likely as men to be depressed. Experts believe genetics play a role: If you have a parent who has struggled with depression, you are more likely to experience it. The cause of the disorder is still unknown, but doctors believe it may be connected to altered brain chemistry. Communication between brain cells that regulate mood may work less efficiently in those with depression, causing an imbalance of the neurotransmitters serotonin, norepinephrine, and dopamine.

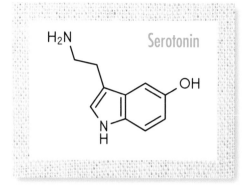

# Types of Depression

Several types of depression exist; physicians can determine which type is present by asking a series of questions. Major depressive disorder lasts for at least two weeks, and can be characterized by the symptoms listed above. Persistent depressive disorder, which was once called dysthymia, is a mild, moderate or severe form of depression that can last for at least two years, with a few days here and there of remission. Bipolar disorder is diagnosed when a person goes through an abnormally high elevated mood for days, and sometimes also has episodes of major depression. Someone with bipolar disorder is more likely to contemplate suicide than those in the general population.

Another type of depression is called seasonal affective disorder and occurs during the winter when less natural light is available and the normal circadian rhythm of the body is disrupted. It's more common farther north where less light is available in winter.

It's important to note that depression is a disorder like other conditions including diabetes, and just like those who suffer from diabetes cannot just snap out of it, neither can those who deal with depressive disorders. Treatment is necessary to help with symptoms and some people may suffer with depressive disorders their entire life.

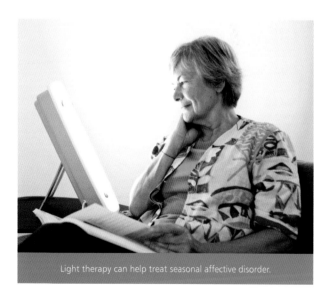

Light therapy can help treat seasonal affective disorder.

# Traditional Depression Treatments

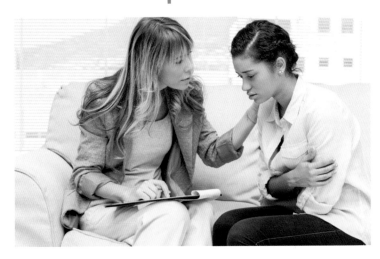

Common treatments for depression include psychotherapy, medication, group therapy, and brain stimulation therapy. With mild to moderate depression, talk therapy can often help. Patients learn to change thoughts and behaviors that contribute to depressed feelings. Therapy can help sufferers work through issues with relationships or unresolved issues.

Exercise can also be a great way to help stave off mild depression, as it increases mood-boosting endorphins, plus helps increase energy and improve sleep. Other depression-busters include maintaining a supportive social circle (whether that be friends and family, support groups, or taking classes at a gym), or even adopting a pet—studies have shown that pet owners have better overall health than those who don't have a furry friend. In addition, light therapy, especially in winter, can be helpful. Light therapy involves sitting near what's called a light therapy box that gives off natural outdoor light. Light therapy likely affects brain chemicals linked to mood and sleep and could stave off symptoms of seasonal depressive disorder as well other types of depression.

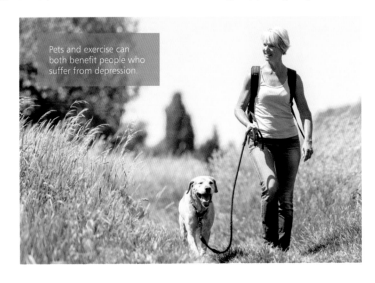

Pets and exercise can both benefit people who suffer from depression.

Medications are also prescribed for those with depression, and often go hand in hand with talk therapy. The most commonly prescribed are called selective serotonin reuptake inhibitors. Newer drugs called serotonin and norepinephrine reuptake inhibitors also are used. Psychiatrists prescribe these drugs in certain dosages, observe the patient's reaction, and determine what the best dosage may be. They may also combine several antidepressant drugs. Some of these drugs have side effects including weight gain, sexual dysfunction, insomnia, and others.

Those suffering from bipolar disorder are given different medications or combinations of medications compared with those who are diagnosed with depressive disorder. These medications also can have side effects, such as poor concentration, drowsiness, hair loss, and weight gain.

It's important to note that it may take several weeks for these medications to take full effect.

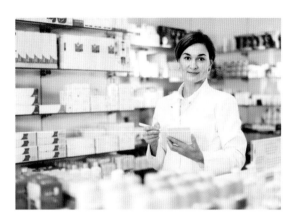

Brain stimulation therapies may be considered if other treatments have not been successful. Electroconvulsive therapy uses an electric current to simulate the brain; it can cause memory loss and other side effects. A new type of brain stimulation uses a magnet instead of an electric current, but some say it's not effective in the long run.

In extreme cases, people suffering from depressive disorders need to be hospitalized, observed, and treated with medication and therapy.

# Depression and CBD

Research has shown that using CBD may help treat depression in a similar way that it can help reduce stress, curb insomnia, and maintain a proper appetite.

The Depression Alliance states that CBD oil helps to significantly improve depressive symptoms and the individual's quality of life, provided the proper dosage is found and it's taken daily. Animal tests showed CBD has similar effects to certain antidepressants. CBD is not a cure for the disorder, but rather treats symptoms just as medications do.

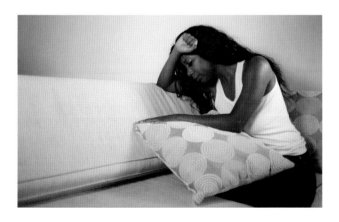

As for bipolar disorder, preliminary tests with CBD show that it likely does not help with the manic stage of the disorder. More studies are being done regarding bipolar depression and CBD usage.

All patients suffering with depressive disorders should talk to their physicians before adding CBD to other prescribed treatments.

# Anxiety

Generalized anxiety disorder affects nearly 7 million Americans. Symptoms include chest pain, heart palpitations, sweating, and the inability to calm down. Other symptoms include constant worrying, being indecisive, and experiencing unwarranted fear of certain people or situations.

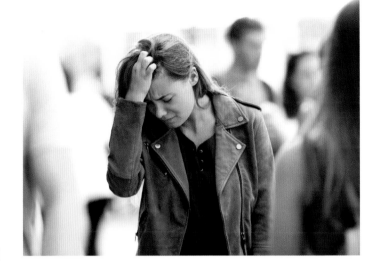

Stressful situations, family history, and different illnesses can cause anxiety. General anxiety disorders can also occur with other mental health problems, for example, depressive disorder, which can make treatment more challenging. In addition, panic disorders and obsessive compulsive disorders are linked to generalized anxiety.

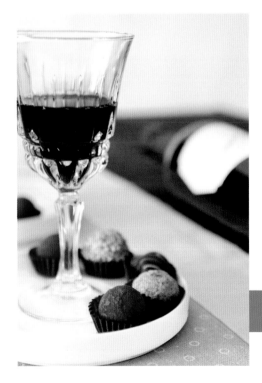

Note that generalized anxiety is different from what are called panic attacks. A panic attack is a sudden onset of fear, which can include an increased heart rate, shortness of breath, and the thoughts you are going to die. These attacks usually last for about 30 minutes. Sugar, alcohol, caffeine, and transfats may trigger panic attacks, according to some experts. Panic attacks may or may not be related to general anxiety disorder.

For all these conditions, though, medication including some antidepressants are used. Talk therapy along with meditation also can help, as well as biofeedback and breathing exercises.

While people often turn to wine and chocolate for comfort, both can act as triggers for panic attacks.

# Anxiety and CBD

Studies using animal models have shown CBD can reduce anxiety; CBD has also been shown to reduce anxiety in patients suffering from social anxiety disorder. In another study, CBD was said to be as effective in treating anxiety compared with several medications used by humans.

CBD was found as a possible deterrent to panic attacks with some people who were facing stressful situations.

Researchers hope to conduct future clinical trials to determine how CBD might affect those with panic disorder, obsessive-compulsive disorder, and social anxiety disorder. Research especially needs to be done to determine dosages and therapeutic rates for these disorders.

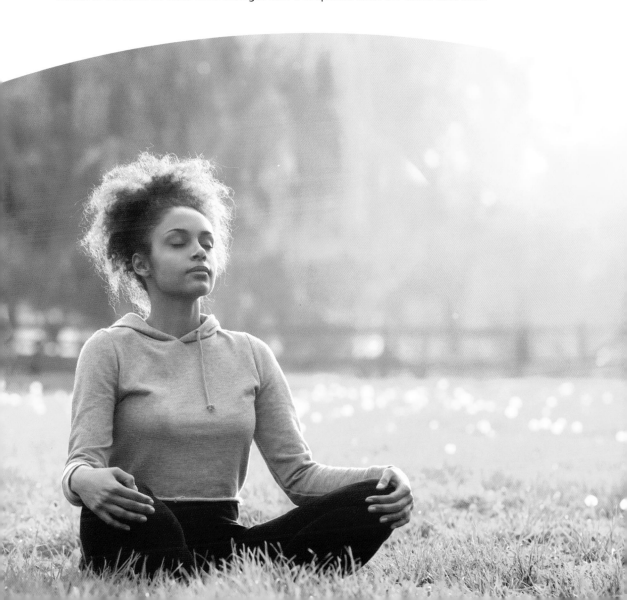

# Diabetes

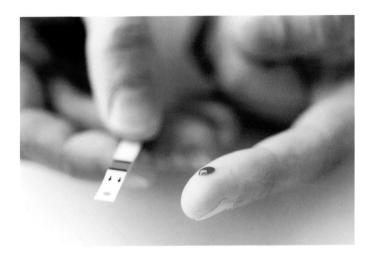

More than 400 million people worldwide suffer from Type 2 diabetes, which is about 95 percent of the population of those with diabetes, with the remaining 5 percent having Type 1 diabetes. In the United States alone, more than 100 million people suffer from either Type 1 or Type 2 diabetes. An estimated 84 million more are prediabetic, meaning they could develop Type 2 diabetes in about five years if nothing is to done to stop it.

In Type 1 diabetes, the body cannot produce insulin, which is needed to move glucose from the bloodstream into cells. Those who contract Type 1 diabetes may have the disease in their family, or their immune system has gone haywire. Children and young adults contract Type 1 diabetes.

With Type 2 diabetes, the body still produces insulin. However, either the body is not able to produce it in the required amount or it is unable to control blood glucose levels.

Developing diabetes has been linked to obesity, genetics, a high sugar diet and ethnicity—African-Americans, Hispanics, and American Indians are more susceptible than other ethnic groups. Those with diabetes can experience life-threatening symptoms such as nerve damage, stroke, vision issues, kidney disease, heart disease, and others. The average diabetic lives 10 to 15 years shorter than someone who does not have the disease.

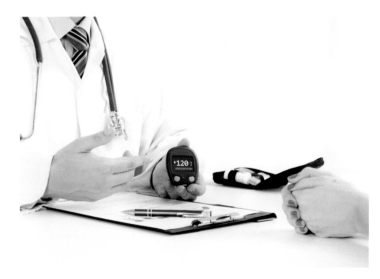

Various tests are available to determine if a person has type 1, type 2 diabetes, or prediabetes. A non-fasting blood test checks your average blood sugar level for several months—higher blood sugar levels indicate prediabetes or diabetes. Fasting blood sugar tests are taken as well, with a level of about 100 mg/dL being normal, and higher than that, indicating possible diabetes. Physicians also administers oral glucose tolerance tests to measure blood sugar levels during the day after the patient is given sugar liquid.

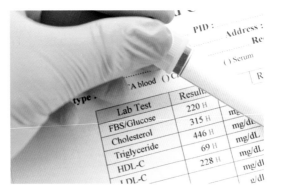

# Diabetes Treatment

Keeping track of glucose levels and eating a proper diet can help diabetics lead a fairly normal life style. Those with Type 1 diabetes learn to administer insulin shots and monitor their glucose levels. Other treatments include a pump that monitors blood glucose and adds insulin when needed. Unfortunately, some of these treatments can be cost-prohibitive for some people.

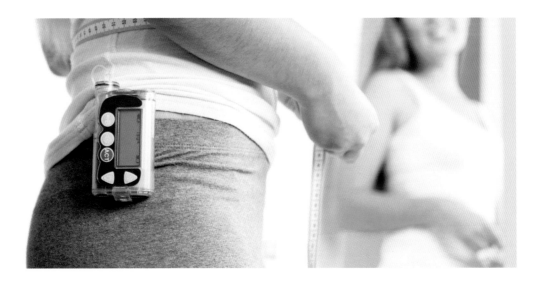

Those with Type 2 diabetes who don't need insulin shots typically are prescribed drugs that help regulate glucose. The drugs can be costly and produce side effects such as diarrhea, yeast infections, nausea, shortness of breath, and low blood pressure. These side effects and their degree of severity can vary among patients.

# Diabetes and CBD

A five-year study has shown that CBD oil may be able to slow or stop the onset of diabetes, so it might be useful for preventing the disease. But once the disease has been diagnosed, CBD oil has not been shown to cure it. Still, studies suggest CBD oil can help with symptoms. For example, diabetics often experience what is called neuropathy or nerve damage, mostly in the hands and feet. It's possible CBD oil may increase the body's level of nerve growth fact and protect the liver from what's called oxidative stress, a contributor to neuropathy.

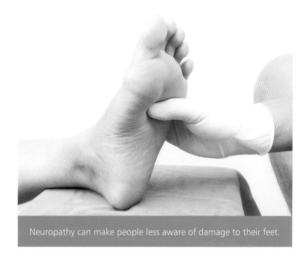

Neuropathy can make people less aware of damage to their feet.

Preliminary studies show that CBD oil may be able to help slow damage to cells in those have who have type 1 diabetes. Work is being done to determine whether CBD can help keep diabetics from getting an eye disorder or developing cardiovascular problems.

Researchers have concluded that using marijuana can help reduce insulin levels in diabetics, but not much research has been done on whether using CBD can do so. Some researchers also think that CBD can help prevent obesity, which can lead to diabetes.

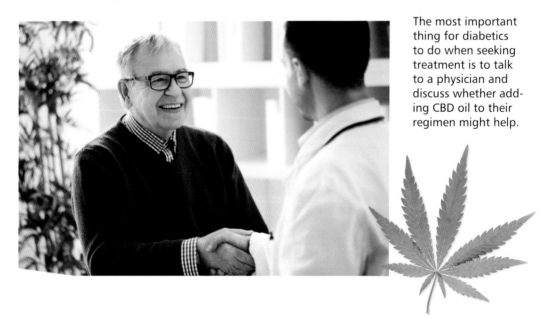

The most important thing for diabetics to do when seeking treatment is to talk to a physician and discuss whether adding CBD oil to their regimen might help.

# Eating Disorders

Obesity and anorexia are two extreme eating disorders—and both may be related to defects in the endocannabinoid system.

Some 30 million Americans suffer from anorexia. While the eating disorder is mostly seen in females, it goes across all ages, races, and genders.

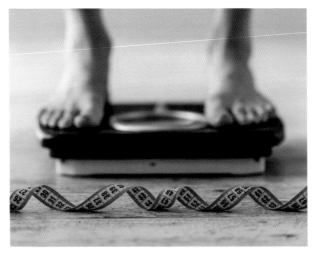

Anorexia is a mental illness in which a person curtails their eating to lose weight—the disease can lead to disability or death. Nearly thirteen percent of sufferers succumb to this disorder, the highest mortality rate of any mental illness.

Research has not been able to name definitively a cause for anorexia, but some contributing factors could be genetics, anxiety, depression, and obsessive-compulsive disorders. Someone with immediate family members who suffer from anorexia is twelve times more likely to develop the disease themselves. A 2011 study published in *Behavioral Neurobiology of Eating* states that the heritable risk of anorexia is twenty-eight to fifty-eight percent.

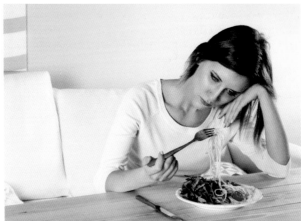

## Anorexia Symptoms

People with anorexia can hide their disease for a long time, but physical symptoms do emerge. These include fatigue, dehydration, thinning hair, dry skin, low blood pressure, dehydration, and major weight loss. Some anorexics also exercise to the point of pure exhaustion.

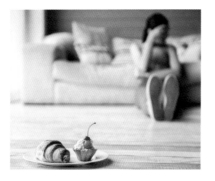

Some patients with anorexia nervosa may binge and purge; this means they eat a lot of food and then vomit or use laxatives and exercise excessively to rid themselves of the calories. This type of binging and purging is different from those suffering from bulimia nervosa. Those patients typically are not underweight and don't stop eating for long periods of time like anorexic patients do.

Anorexia can worsen, causing osteoporosis, seizures, abnormal blood counts, and eventually hospitalization.

# Anorexia Treatments

No specific anti-anorexia medications are available. Instead patients are advised to seek a counselor and take antidepressants. Treatment may also include nutrition education and health monitoring, as well as observation in a hospital.

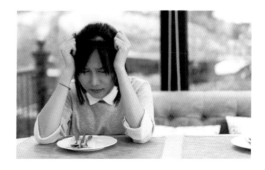

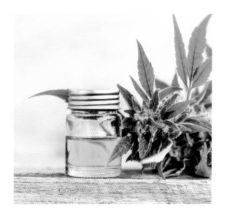

# Anorexia and CBD

Medical marijuana, where it is legal, is used to treat anorexia. But researchers also think CBD can help.

One small study in Belgium discovered that those with eating disorders also have an imbalance in their endocannabinoid systems. Since CBD can react with receptors within the body related to this system, it may be able to help those with eating disorders, without the psychoactive effects of THC.

Some mental health advocates think that using CBD with talk therapy can help those with anorexia by relieving stress and working with the body's endocannabinoid system.

Some experts say CBD regulates the appetite and helps your body use food properly.

Anecdotal evidence shows that those suffering from bulimia may benefit from vaping CBD to reduce anxiety, which can decrease the desire to binge.

# Obesity

Obesity is a popular topic in the 21st century, and there's concern that the population of people who are obese is growing. Someone is considered obese when they have so much body fat that it negatively impacts their health. Physicians use body mass index to determine if a person is overweight or obese. A body mass index between 25 and 29.9 signals overweight; one that is more than 30 points to obesity. The body mass index is determined by using a formula based on height and weight.

Leading a sedentary lifestyle, eating too many calories, not getting enough sleep, and ingesting fructose, taking certain medications, and family history are linked to obesity. Losing weight and keeping it off involves increasing physical activity, changing how and when you eat, and modifying behaviors. Some patients may also be given medication and others might have surgery.

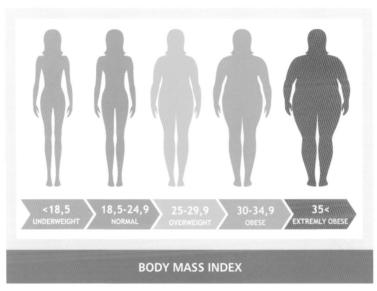

| <18,5 UNDERWEIGHT | 18,5-24,9 NORMAL | 25-29,9 OVERWEIGHT | 30-34,9 OBESE | 35< EXTREMLY OBESE |

**BODY MASS INDEX**

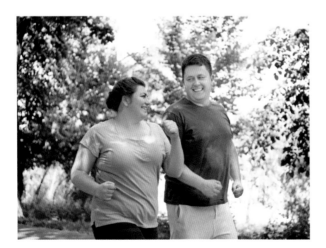

# Obesity and CBD

One study shows CBD might be helpful in treating obesity. Researchers studied the relationship between CBD and brown fat, a type of cell that burns calories rather than storing them. Some conjecture that CBD could be used to "create" more brown fat or replace what's called white fat, the not-so-good-fat, with brown fat. Much more research needs to be done on obesity and CBD.

# Epilepsy

The fourth most common neurological disorder, epilepsy is characterized by unpredictable and recurrent seizures due to a surge of electrical activity in the brain. This surge of activity causes a disruption in the messages sent by the brain to other areas of the body. The disorder affects 3.4 million Americans, including around 470,000 children. For about one third of those people, available treatments are ineffective. The cause of epilepsy is often completely unknown, although occasionally it can be a result of brain trauma or a family history of the disease.

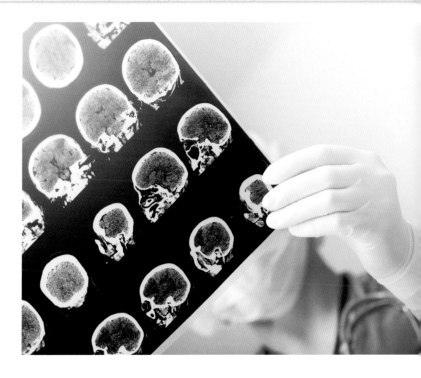

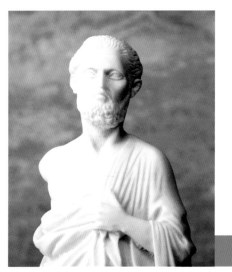

Hippocrates

Hippocrates of Kos, the Greek physician who is a seminal figure in the history of medicine, was one of the first notable people to reject the popular antiquarian view that epilepsy was a sacred disease caused by the gods. The ancient Greeks thought of epilepsy as a type of spiritual possession that they associated with both genius and divine intervention. It was often associated with the moon goddess, Selene, who would afflict people with the sacred disease if she was not happy with them. Hippocrates later disputed such assumptions in his work *On the Sacred Disease*, where he claimed that epilepsy was not divine in origin, but stemmed from a treatable disease of the brain.

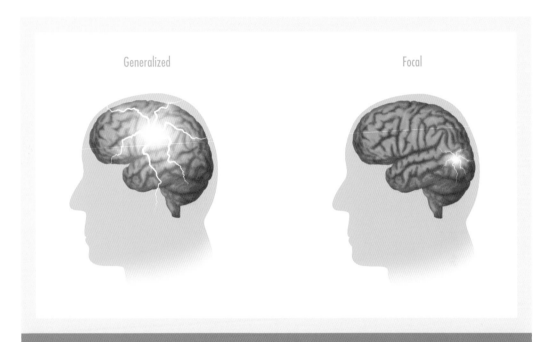

Generalized

Focal

**TYPES OF EPILEPSY**

Some of the symptoms of generalized and focal onset seizures are similar—both can result in motor symptoms like jerking movements, muscles becoming either weak and limp or rigid and tense, and muscle twitching and spasms. Generalized onset seizures can also have non-motor symptoms called absence seizures. Absence seizures do not cause the dramatic muscle twitches often associated with epilepsy, but rather are categorized by lapses in awareness and staring. They are more common in children than adults, and can be so brief that they are sometimes mistaken for daydreaming.

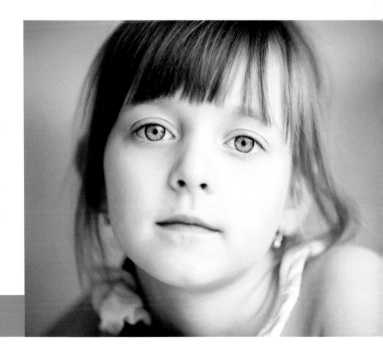

Absence seizures can be mistaken for daydreaming.

Focal onset seizures can have non-motor symptoms as well, which manifest as changes in sensation, emotions, thinking, or autonomic functions such as waves of heat or cold, goosebumps, or a racing heart. There are two types of focal onset seizures: focal onset aware and focal onset impaired awareness. Focal aware seizures often affect the temporal lobes and precede more traumatic generalized seizures. Those who suffer from focal awareness seizures stay conscious. Focal impaired seizures often affect larger sections of the hemisphere and cause the sufferer to lose consciousness.

Generalized seizures affect both hemispheres of the brain and impair consciousness. There are many types of seizures that are categorized under the generalized seizure umbrella, including absence seizures, myoclonic seizures, clonic seizures, tonic-clonic seizures, and atonic seizures.

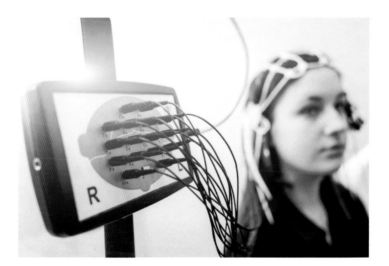

An electroencephalogram can monitor the activity of your brains waves and can help in the diagnosis of epilepsy and epileptic seizures. The test also can be used to determine whether the seizure a patient is experiencing is a focal onset or generalized onset seizure.

# Epilepsy Treatment

Epilepsy can be a very disruptive disorder, causing issues with school or work, and affecting a person's ability to drive or live alone. Those with epilepsy are more susceptible to depression and anxiety, can have learning disabilities, may have problems sleeping,

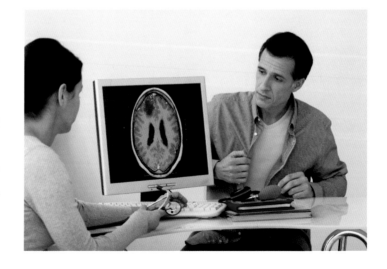

and are at risk for falls and injuries. There is no cure for the disorder, but sufferers have several treatment options. Anti-epileptic drugs are usually the first course of action, but if those don't work, surgery may be a possibility. Surgery is especially helpful for those whose seizures are a result of benign brain tumors or structural defects. Another option is an implantable neuromodulation device. These devices use small electrical currents to signal the malfunctioning nerve cells to work correctly.

Anti-epileptic drugs come with a laundry list of possible side effects, including dizziness, sleep issues, slurred speech, double vision, weight gain, loss of bone density, rashes, and memory problems. Some people find they simply cannot tolerate the side effects of the drugs. Plus one-third of epilepsy sufferers have difficulty finding a treatment that works.

Aside from anticonvulsant medications and surgery for treating epilepsy, some studies have shown a ketogenic diet might reduce the amount of seizures one experiences. Basically, a ketogenic diet consists of high fats and low carbohydrates said to lower blood sugar and insulin levels. Many types of ketogenic diets exist, so it's best to speak with a dietitian or physician.

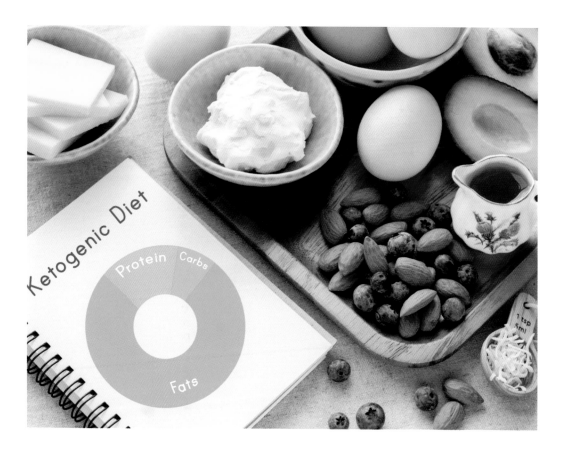

# Epilepsy and CBD

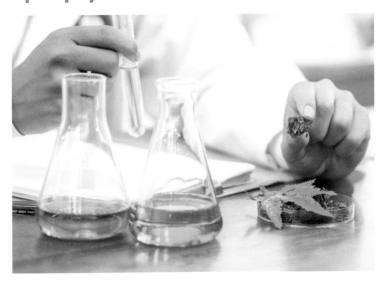

The most exciting advance in epilepsy treatment came when in June 2018, the FDA approved the drug Epidiolex, an oral solution of CBD, to treat seizures that occur with two rare and severe forms of epilepsy called Lennox-Gastaut syndrome and Dravet syndrome, in patients ages two and older. Epidiolex was not created with synthetics but specifically comes from the Cannabis plant.

Three double-blind studies were conducted, involving 516 patients with either one of the syndromes. Those given Epidiolex and other medications experienced fewer seizures than those in the control group.

Research has shown some promise in using a product that has high CBD and low THC. One strain known as Charlotte's Web was named after a five-year-old girl named Charlotte Figi, whose severe epilepsy was brought under control using the strain in a concentrated oil.

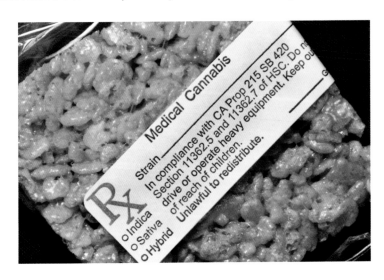

A high CBD strain seems to be key in treating the disorder, as the cannabinoid might be effective in reducing seizures. Plus, a low-THC strain ensures that those with epilepsy can control their seizures while still remaining clear-headed throughout their day.

In a 2016 study, children with epilepsy used high-CBD oils. Almost seventy percent were shown to have 50 percent fewer seizures and some of them, about fifteen percent, were seizure free. Some experienced side effects including tiredness and diarrhea.

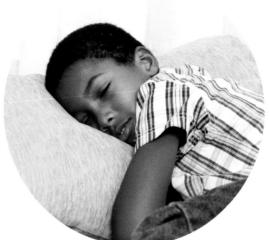

Oils and tinctures are popular consumption methods, although for adults, smoking or vaporization may be used for more immediate relief. But the advantage for using an oil or tincture is that a very precise dosage can be used—once the effective dose is found, it is easy to continue dosing the correct amount. Be aware, however, that the FDA has not approved use of CBD oil for any type of seizures, and that Epidiolex has undergone clinical studies to treat only two rare types of epilepsy.

In May 2018, Dr. Orrin Devinsky, director of Langone's Comprehensive Epilepsy Center in New York City, said it was not clear whether CBD could help those with the more common types of epilepsy. He said small clinical trials showed no benefit to people who experience focal epilepsy.

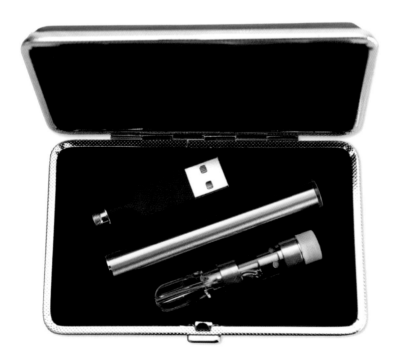

# Fibromyalgia

Fibromyalgia is one of the most common bone and muscle disorders, and is characterized by pain in joints and muscles throughout the body. Fatigue, which can be debilitating in some patients, is also common. Other symptoms include migraines, restless leg syndrome, anxiety, issues with thinking, numbness in various parts of the body, and irritable bowel syndrome.

Some physicians believe fibromyalgia is caused by a problem in the way in which pain signals from your nerves get processed, but no real cause has been identified. Those more susceptible to getting fibromyalgia include women, people with anxiety or depression, people who have other diseases that cause pain, and those who suffer from post-traumatic stress disorder. Genetics may play a role, and certain types of infections also can trigger fibromyalgia. In one case, Lyme disease may have been a contributing cause.

Those with fibromyalgia sometimes think they have tendinitis or arthritis—but the pain in those cases is often more localized. With fibromyalgia, patients typically feel the pain throughout the body.

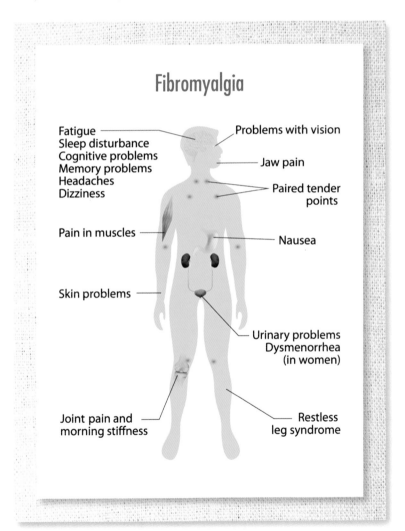

Fibromyalgia

Fatigue
Sleep disturbance
Cognitive problems
Memory problems
Headaches
Dizziness

Problems with vision

Jaw pain

Paired tender points

Pain in muscles

Nausea

Skin problems

Urinary problems
Dysmenorrhea
(in women)

Joint pain and
morning stiffness

Restless
leg syndrome

Before it was called fibromyalgia, the medical community referred to the disorder as fibrositis, a condition in which soft tissue pain moved throughout the body. The term was likely coined in the early 1900s.

Physicians typically rule out other illnesses by ordering blood tests and X-rays. If none of those are positive, the physician asks a series of questions and works out a treatment plan with the patient. In addition, patients often have painful nodules, especially in the shoulder and neck, that can limit movement.

No cure has been found.

# Treatments

Physicians often suggest fibromyalgia patients use over-the-counter and prescribed medications to reduce pain and ease depression and anxiety. Combining medication with increased exercise, stress management, and eating well also can positively affect a patient suffering with fibromyalgia. Stronger pain killers including opioids can lead to addiction, and often are not recommended for prolonged use by fibromyalgia patients.

Physicians also advise low-impact exercise such as walking, yoga, and tai chi. Other treatments may include massage and acupuncture.

One program at the Mayo Clinic works with patients to stop using pain and sleep medication and work on managing their pain including physical therapy, biofeedback, exercise, counseling, and other techniques.

Some sufferers have turned to an herb called kratom, obtained from outside the United States. Kratom is touted to relieve pain and anxiety associated with fibromyalgia. The FDA has warned that using kratom can have minor to life-threatening side effects, and can be addictive. Kratom has also been linked to salmonella by the FDA.

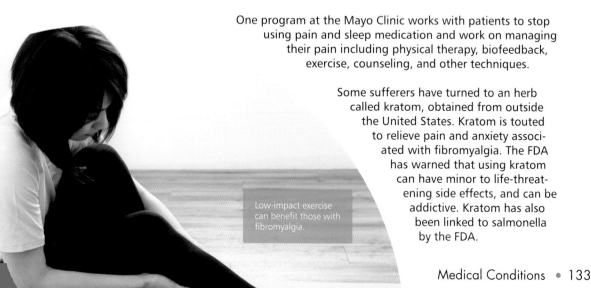

Low-impact exercise can benefit those with fibromyalgia.

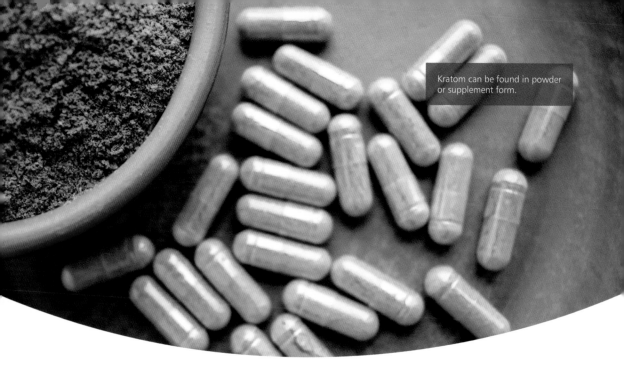

Kratom can be found in powder or supplement form.

# Fibromyalgia and CBD

Researchers have discovered that CBD can reduce some symptoms of fibromyalgia, but that it does not work with everyone. They think that CBD may interrupt pain signals in the body. One study has led researchers to consider whether those with a weakened endocannabinoid system may develop fibromyalgia, and whether CBD might put the system back in balance. Debate also exists about the concentration of CBD required to be effective in treating symptoms.

Carrie Anton, an online blogger for *Fibromyalgia News Today*, who suffers with fibromyalgia, wrote that after using CBD for three days, she was able to sleep better and experience less pain and anxiety.

Dr. Ginevra Liptan, a physician who developed fibromyalgia in medical school, said though no real studies can point to CBD helping the disorder in humans, she has found it useful for herself. She said CBD has helped with joint and muscle pain and reduced her anxiety. She also said some of her patients find relief from CBD, while others don't. Dr. Liptan is the founder and medical director of the Frida Center for Fibromyalgia.

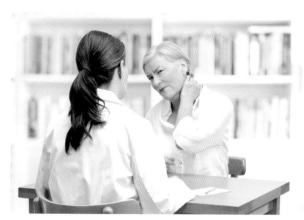

# Glaucoma

Some three million Americans have glaucoma, which is the leading cause of blindness in the United States. Ten percent of them have some vision loss even with proper treatment. Blindness as a result or the disease is more common in African-Americans compared with Caucasians.

Glaucoma is related to the fluid pressure in the eye. When it rises above normal levels, it could be the start of glaucoma. Causes are mostly unknown although diabetes, cataracts, and tumors could lead to glaucoma. Eye injuries, old age, and certain other conditions also can lead to glaucoma.

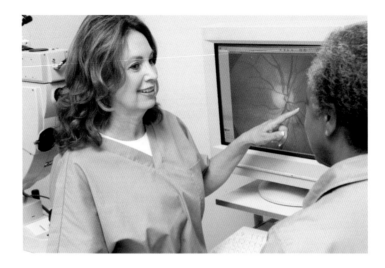

Several types of glaucoma exist. Open-angle glaucoma is the most common, and affects about ninety-five percent of people with the disease. With this type, the drainage canal in the eyes aren't working properly; medication can help and the condition severity increases very slowly.

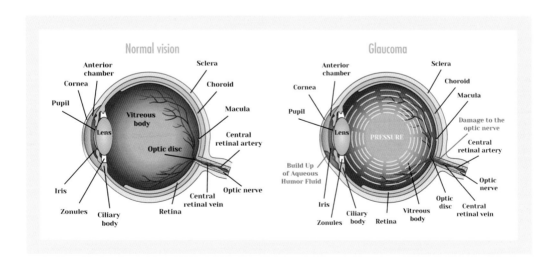

Angle-closure glaucoma is rare and involves rapid rising of eye pressure. Pain, headaches, blurred vision, and nausea are some of the symptoms. Treatment for this type of glaucoma often involves surgery.

To determine if a patient has glaucoma, eye doctors can administer several tests. One of them measures the pressure of the eye. Others take pictures of the shape and color of the optic nerve and the angle in the eye where the iris and cornea connect, as well as the thickness of the cornea. A field of vision test that measures peripheral vision also is given. Peripheral vision is often the first part of the vision that decreases with glaucoma patients.

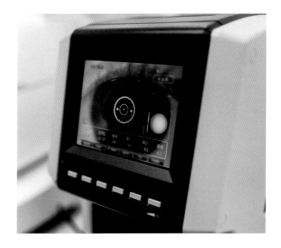

Physicians recommend having your eyes tested between six months and a few years depending on your age and risk factors.

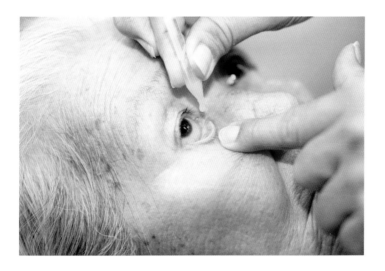

# Glaucoma Treatments

With open angle glaucoma, physicians prescribe eye drops that work to decrease fluid production or help the fluids leave the eye. Side effects include low blood pressure, depression, and fatigue. If medicine doesn't help, laser surgery can be tried. A laser, a beam of intense light, is sent to the eye to drain fluid and open clogged areas. It may take several weeks to notice if it's worked. Various other types of surgeries can be tried if the first type doesn't work.

For more advanced cases, drainage implants and other in-hospital surgeries may be warranted—glaucoma surgery increases the chances of getting cataracts and it can't restore any eyesight that's been lost.

# Glaucoma and CBD

No cure has been found for glaucoma, and no large scale clinical trials have been done to determine if CBD can help with glaucoma.

Studies have shown that cannabis—with high strains of THC—can lower ocular pressure. However, you'd need to consume the THC every few hours, otherwise the effects are gone. That's not a viable option.

But perhaps CBD can help. One study in 1979 showed that CBD taken by 16 patients with open-angle glaucoma helped lower their eye pressure. But how much to administer and how to administer it are questions that need to be answered before it's even considered for use to treat glaucoma. One study, for example, showed that eye pressure was actually raised when a patient was given 40 milligrams of CBD. Another study showed that if the proper dose is administered topically, CBD may decrease ocular pressure. Much more needs to be done to determine whether CBD may help with glaucoma. For the time being, if you're taking prescribed medication such as eye drops for glaucoma, speak to your physician before adding CBD, and have your eye pressure check regularly.

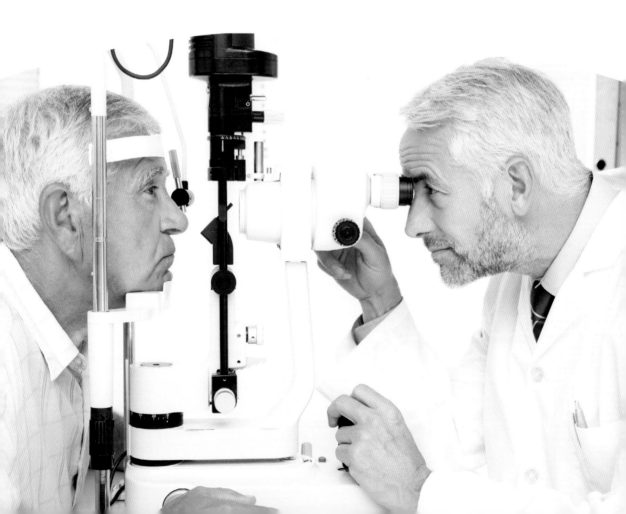

# Heart Disease

More than 80 million Americans suffer from heart disease, or as it is sometimes called, cardiovascular disease. The term refers to conditions that affect the heart such as coronary artery disease, arrhythmia (an irregular heart beat), and birth defects. Heart disease can be linked to narrow blood vessels, which can cause heart attack, stroke, and chest pain. Overall, heart disease is the leading cause of death in the United States.

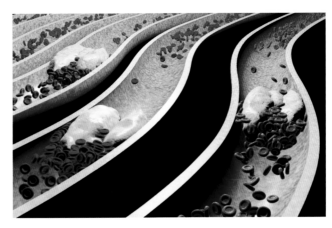

Symptoms vary depending on the type of heart disease, and they may differ between men and women.

Heart disease symptoms depend on what type of heart disease you have.

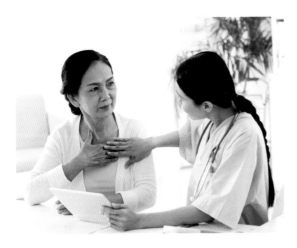

If the disease is in your blood vessels, it's called atherosclerotic disease. Men typically experience chest pain while women may experience nausea, fatigue, and shortness of breath. In addition, the disease can produce a pain or numbness in legs or arms, as well as in the neck, jaw, throat, upper abdomen, or back. People often are not diagnosed with the disease until after they have a heart attack, stroke, or major chest pain.

Those with abnormal heart beats might experience fluttering in the chest, a slow or racing heartbeat, chest pain, dizziness, and lightheadedness, including fainting.

Serious heart defects are typically found soon after a person is born. Symptoms include blue- or gray-colored skin, swelling in the legs or abdomen, and difficulties breathing.

Other heart diseases can be caused by an infection. Symptoms include cough, skin rash, swelling in the legs or abdomen, fatigue, and shortness of breath.

A damaged heart valve can also lead to heart disease. Symptoms include fatigue, shortness of breath, chest pain, and fainting.

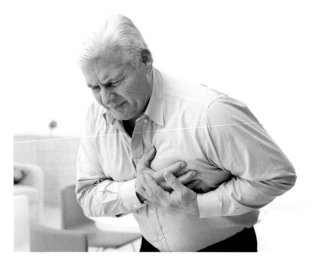

Since many of the symptoms can occur in different types of heart disease, getting a diagnosis is important. Medical care specialists recommend going to the emergency room if you have chest pain, shortness of breath, and fainting spells.

The risk for getting heart disease is higher in elderly people, those with a family history of the disease, smokers, those who have been treated with certain cancer drugs, high blood pressure, a diet high in bad fats, diabetes, obesity, high cholesterol, stress, depression, lack of exercise, and poor hygiene.

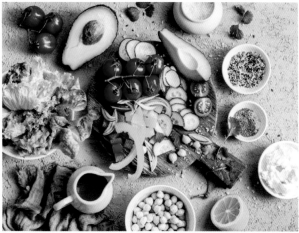

Not all heart disease, for example, a birth defect, can be prevented. But heart specialists stress that eating a good diet, not smoking, controlling high blood pressure and cholesterol, exercising nearly every day, managing stress, and keeping a healthy weight, are all protectants from developing heart disease. Getting your cholesterol and blood pressure checked regularly also can be preventive medicine.

Physicians administer various tests to determine if you have heart disease and what type you might have. These include blood tests and chest X-rays as well as an electrocardiogram, which measures your heart's rhythm, and an ultrasound, which shows images of your heart's structure.

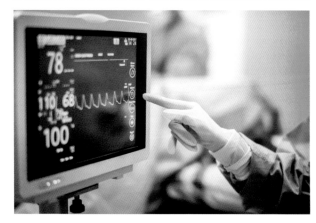

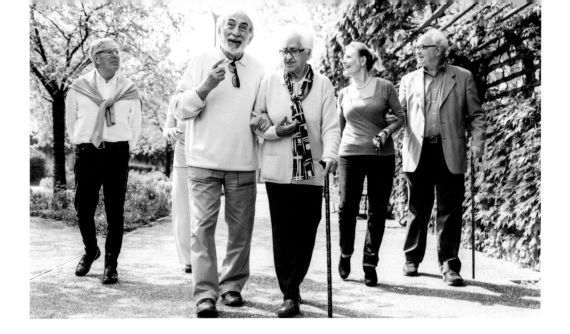

# Treatment

Physicians often recommend lifestyle changes to treat heart disease; they also prescribe medications such as blood thinners. If that doesn't work, medical procedures or surgery might be recommended. Surgery runs the gamut from replacement of heart valves to a heart transplant.

# Heart Disease and CBD

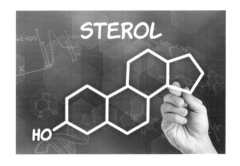

One study done in Great Britain showed that CBD can reduce tension on blood vessel walls; another showed that CBD might be a preventive tactic, since it contains a high amount of sterols, which are said to reduce heart disease risk. Sterols are natural compounds found in plants. Research has shown that plant sterols can lower what's called bad cholesterol. In actuality, a sterol in a plant is very similar to cholesterol found in animals. Since sterols and cholesterol are chemically similar, the sterols are said to be able to block cholesterol from being absorbed by the intestines, and in turn, lower LDL in the blood. LDL is a low-density protein that can clog arteries.

Animal studies have also shown that CBD can reduce blood pressure, leaving some physicians to wonder if medications containing CBD could someday replace current high blood pressure drugs. The door seems to be opening wider for more studies regarding CBD and heart disease, including its potential to prevent it.

# Huntington's Disease

Huntington's disease and Parkinson's disease both affect the part of the brain that involves movement. But each are different in the age group they affect and other factors.

Huntington's disease affects younger people compared with Parkinson's, and is linked to genetics and other factors. This fatal disorder causes nerve cells in the brain to break down so that the person's physical and mental abilities decline drastically.

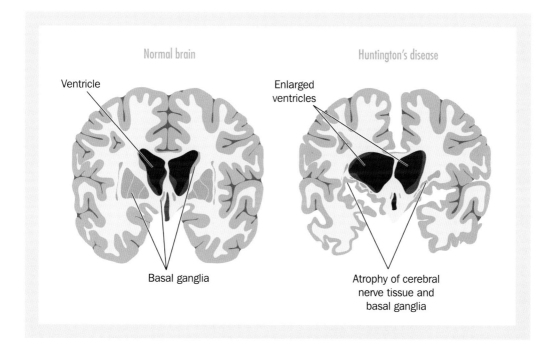

Huntington's has been described as having the symptoms of Alzheimer's and Parkinson's disease combined.

There's no known cure, and every child of a parent with this disease has a 50/50 chance of having the gene that causes it, according to the Huntington's Diseases Society of America. Roughly 30,000 Americans show symptoms of Huntingon's disease, with almost that many having the potential to contract the disease, according to the society.

Patients start experiencing symptoms when they are between 30 and 50 years old. Symptoms include depression, personality changes, unsteady gait, slurred speech, weight loss, difficulty in swallowing, involuntary movements; and eventually the inability to walk and talk. The patient usually dies from complications of the disease including pneumonia and heart failure. Researchers discovered the gene that causes the disease in 1993, and they are working toward a cure. A blood test can determine if a person with Huntingon's disease in the family has the positive gene that could lead to them contracting the disease.

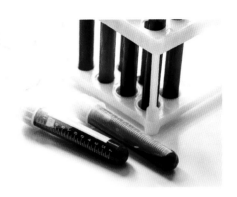

The disease is diagnosed based on physical, neurological, and psychiatric exams and family history.

# Treatment

Nothing can cure Huntington's disease, but medications can help with some symptoms including movement challenges and mental issues. Some drugs treat some symptoms, but make others worse. One of the common symptoms called chorea, which involves irregular and abrupt movements, is being treated with one medication that can lessen the symptoms. A few other medicines not designated for Huntington's disease have been prescribed in hopes of helping the patient. Some antipsychotic drugs are used to reduce chorea and irritability.

Psychotherapy, speech therapy, physical therapy, and occupational therapy, also can help lessen symptoms.

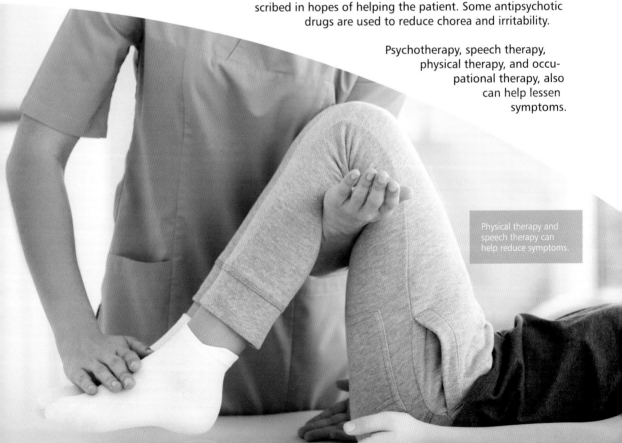

Physical therapy and speech therapy can help reduce symptoms.

# Huntington's Disease and CBD

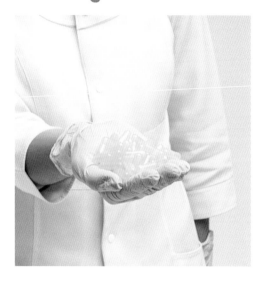

Studies are mixed, but most point to CBD not having an effect on treating Huntington's disease. One study tested patients with the disease and gave them either CBD or a placebo and found no significant differences in symptoms in both sets of patients.

However, some researchers say that CBD has antioxidant properties that might offer relief from some symptoms of Huntington's disease. A British pharmaceutical company developed a spray called Sativex, which contains CBD and has been said to help patients with multiple sclerosis. They think CBD may also help treat Huntington's disease and plan to do more research on the subject. As of this writing, Sativex had not been approved by the FDA. Some researchers think a higher concentration of THC in CBD may be able to help Huntington's disease patients.

One study done in Spain concluded the use of cannabinoids can improve fine motor skills of those with Huntington's disease as well as curb their irritability.

A Canadian patient offered anecdotal evidence that CBD helped her counteract some symptoms; for example, by vaping with CBD, she said her hand was not moving as uncontrollably as it was before.

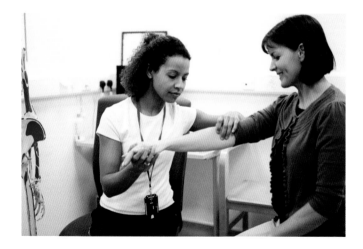

The mother of a Canadian patient who acquired Huntington's disease as a juvenile and is now confined to a wheelchair reported that giving her daughter CBD oil has improved her speech and her ability to eat without choking. She sometimes can stand and has stopped shaking, according to her mother. The oil she's using has a very low THC content.

Overall, though, the main belief in the United States is that CBD has no effect on reducing the symptoms or course of Huntington's disease.

# Inflammatory Bowel Diseases

Some 1.6 million Americans suffer from inflammatory bowel diseases, including ulcerative colitis or Crohn's disease. Inflammatory bowel disease should not be confused with inflammatory bowel syndrome, a disorder affecting muscle contractions of the colon and not linked to an inflammation of the intestines, as are Crohn's and colitis.

Ulcerative colitis is a chronic disease of the large intestine, also known as the colon, in which the lining of the colon becomes inflamed and develops tiny open sores, or ulcers, that produce pus and mucous. The combination of inflammation and ulceration can cause abdominal discomfort and frequent emptying of the colon.

Ulcerative colitis is the result of an abnormal response by your body's immune system. Crohn's disease can affect any part of the gastrointestinal tract, but ulcerative colitis affects only the colon. Additionally, while Crohn's disease can affect all layers of the bowel wall, ulcerative colitis only affects the colon's lining.

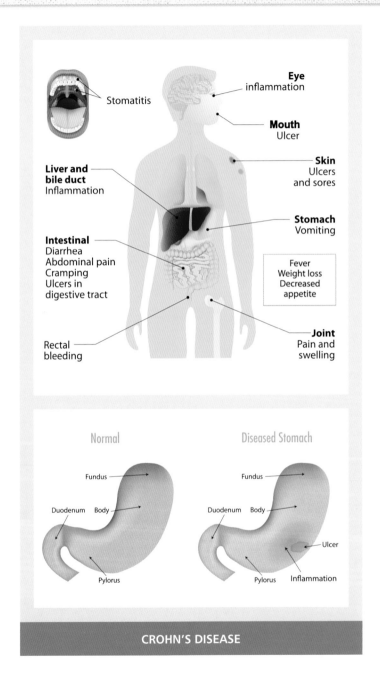

Stomatitis

**Eye** inflammation

**Mouth** Ulcer

**Skin** Ulcers and sores

**Liver and bile duct** Inflammation

**Stomach** Vomiting

**Intestinal** Diarrhea Abdominal pain Cramping Ulcers in digestive tract

Fever Weight loss Decreased appetite

**Joint** Pain and swelling

Rectal bleeding

Normal

Diseased Stomach

Fundus

Duodenum   Body

Pylorus

Fundus

Duodenum   Body

Ulcer

Pylorus   Inflammation

**CROHN'S DISEASE**

# Colitis Symptoms

Half of patients with ulcerative colitis experience mild to severe symptoms, including constant diarrhea, abdominal pain, blood in the stool, as well as loss of appetite, weight loss and fatigue.

The symptoms can come and go often with months, if not longer, of remission.

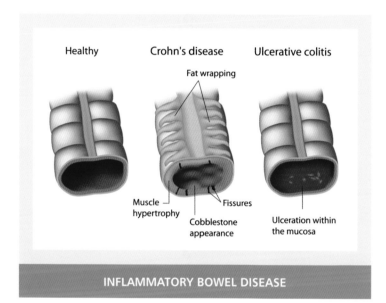

Healthy     Crohn's disease     Ulcerative colitis

Fat wrapping

Muscle hypertrophy    Fissures

Cobblestone appearance

Ulceration within the mucosa

**INFLAMMATORY BOWEL DISEASE**

The cause of ulcerative colitis is unknown, although some studies show that genetics, environmental factors and immune system deficiencies might contribute. Some research also points to a viral or bacterial infection in the colon.

Physicians make a diagnosis based on medical history, an examination, and blood and stool tests. Other more invasive tests include an examination of the colon via medical instruments inserted into the anus.

# Colitis Treatments

Medication to reduce inflammation is one of many ways to lessen the symptoms of colitis. Patients are also given dietary and lifestyle suggestions to keep the disease at bay, and often are restricted from eating dairy products. In about one-fourth to one-third of the patients, surgery may also be an option. The surgery may involve removing the colon and rectum and inserting a device in the skin from which wastes get emptied. Newer surgeries today often can be done without having to insert a device into the skin.

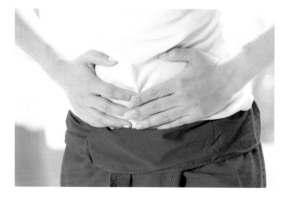

# Crohn's Disease Symptoms

Crohn's disease can affect any part of the digestive tract, although it most commonly attacks the end of the small intestine and beginning of the large intestine. The disease can affect one area while leaving another alone, causing patches of diseased intestine between healthy parts. In a normal gastrointestinal tract, friendly bacteria are present that help aid in digestion—the immune system knows not to attack these harmless bugs. But in the case of Crohn's disease, the bacteria are mistakenly seen as invaders, and the immune system responds, resulting in inflammation. Eventually, the inflammation becomes chronic, leading to thickened intestinal walls, ulcerations, and unpleasant symptoms.

These can include persistent diarrhea, blood in the stools, abdominal cramps and pain, and an urgent need to use the bathroom. Loss of appetite, fatigue, and low energy are also common.

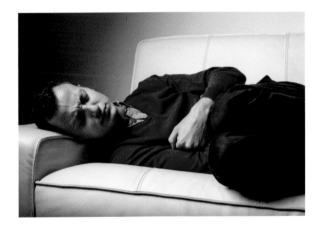

As a chronic disease, Crohn's can disrupt sufferers' lives in multiple ways. The need to always be near a bathroom can mean fewer social activities and result in isolation from friends or family. About half of sufferers miss an average of twenty-six days of work per year. Those who suffer from the disease often worry about job security—many even hide their condition from their employer, fearing it will cost them their job or promotions. The unpredictability of sudden flare-ups can cause constant stress—which, ironically, is thought to be a possible trigger for flare-ups.

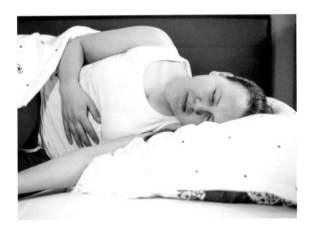

The causes of Crohn's are not well understood, but researchers believe a combination of genetics and environmental factors play a role.

As with colitis, physicians make a diagnosis based on medical history, an examination, and blood and stool tests as well as an examination of the colon via medical instruments inserted into the anus. With Crohn's disease, a physician may also perform small intestinal imaging in which the patient drinks a liquid and has X-rays taken to view what's happening inside the intestine.

# Crohn's Disease Treatment

Treatment for this disease can often include many different medications, such as anti-inflammatory drugs, corticosteroids, immune system modifiers, antibiotics, and nutritional supplements. Surgery is an unfortunate necessity for up to seventy-five percent of Crohn's patients, and can consist of removing the diseased parts of the intestines and joining healthy ends together. While this surgery can help people remain symptom-free for years, it does not cure the disease, and Crohn's may eventually return.

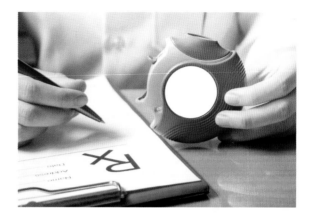

# Leaky Gut Syndrome

Leaky gut is a condition in which the thin, mucus digestive barrier in our stomach stops working correctly. The mucus serves as a way to make sure nutrients are absorbed and to keep undigested food particles and waste products from leaking into the bloodstream and the rest of the body. Illness, inflammation, and allergies can cause leaky gut syndrome. Symptoms include migraines, irritable bowel syndrome, fatigue, and even eczema. This syndrome can be connected to inflammatory bowel disease, Crohn's disease and irritable bowel syndrome.

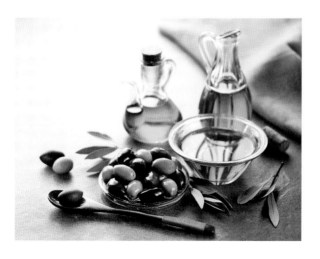

# Leaky Gut Treatment

Nutritionists advise changing the diet by getting rid of gluten, dairy, soy, refined sugar, caffeine, and alcohol, while adding healthy fats such as olive oil. They also recommend taking supplements such as digestive enzymes and glutamine.

# Crohn's, Colitis, Leaky Gut, and CBD

While neither Crohn's nor colitis has a cure, studies are beginning to show that cannabis can be an effective way to alleviate some of the symptoms of these diseases. A 2015 study showed that Crohn's patients had fewer and less severe symptoms after being put on a CBD regimen. A laboratory study showed that rats with induced colitis showed reduced inflammation in the colon after being treated with CBD.

One 2016 study showed that by blocking a certain enzyme in the body, inflammation in the colon might be suppressed. CBD oil has been shown to block that specific enzyme, and someday CBD could be used in new drugs that counteract the symptoms of inflammatory bowel disease.

Preliminary studies have shown that CBD may be able to improve leaky gut syndrome. Although research is still new, some speculate that CBD could help with a variety of digestive issues.

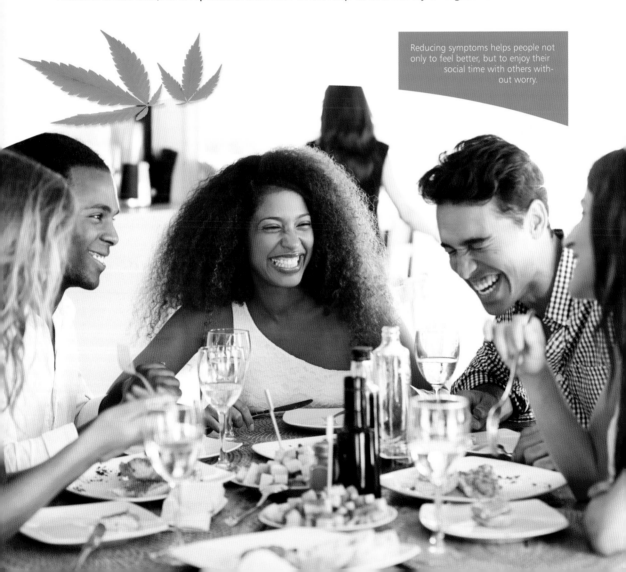

Reducing symptoms helps people not only to feel better, but to enjoy their social time with others without worry.

# Insomnia

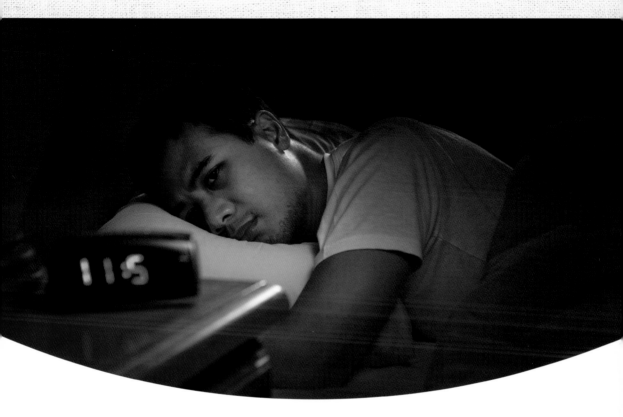

Few things are as frustrating as feeling tired and exhausted but being unable to sleep. You lie down in a nice, comfy bed at the end of the day, close your eyes, and … stay awake for hours. This maddening condition is insomnia, and it is defined as having difficulty falling asleep or staying asleep, even when you have ample opportunity to do so. Approximately 70 million Americans suffer from insomnia or another sleep disorder.

Acute insomnia affects all of us now and then. It can happen when we're worrying about an upcoming event, like a final exam or a big work presentation, or feeling distressed over bad news or events. Between thirty and forty percent of Americans report experiencing acute insomnia each year, but usually, this sort of sleep disruption resolves quickly, without the need for any treatment.

But chronic insomnia, which affects between ten and fifteen percent of Americans, occurs much more often—at least three nights per week, lasting at least three months. Causes can include a change in environment, work schedules, poor sleeping habits, or certain medications. Medical conditions like chronic pain, acid reflux, asthma, or Parkinson's disease can also affect sleep.

# Complications of Insomnia

Those who suffer from insomnia often wake up earlier than they'd like and experience fatigue and sleepiness during the day. They may also feel irritable and anxious, have difficulty concentrating, and endure headaches and gastrointestinal issues. Even worse, a person with insomnia may be particularly uncoordinated and accident-prone in their sleep-deprived state, putting them at higher risk for injuries and making driving and certain other tasks more dangerous than usual.

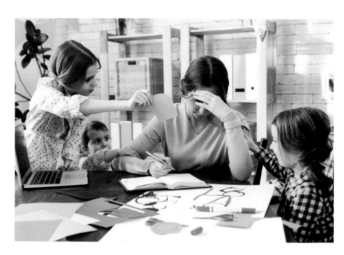

# Treatments

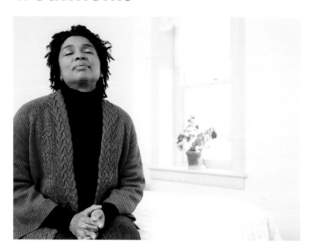

Relaxation techniques such as breathing exercises and meditation can be effective in treating insomnia. Another method is called stimulus control, in which persons are told to only be in the bedroom when it's time to sleep, and to get out of bed if awake for more than 20 minutes. Cognitive behavioral therapy also is considered. It helps people understand their fears about sleeping and change them into positive thoughts. Prescription and over-the-counter drugs are available to help with sleep. Speaking with your physician about what's best for you is recommended.

Some people who suffer from insomnia say that melatonin, a hormone that regulates sleep patterns, helps. Melatonin levels rise substantially at night time, helping the body relax and prepare for sleep. Melatonin is considered a dietary supplement and can be purchased over the counter. Using high dosages is not recommended with melatonin.

# Insomnia and CBD oil

Studies on whether CBD oil can help with sleep are somewhat contradictory. In one study done on rats, those treated with CBD had more and better sleep compared with those who weren't. So the possibility exists that CBD oil could improve your sleep.

However, one study found CBD to provide good sleep the first few hours after taking it and then later causing wakefulness. Some people have anecdotally reported that taking CBD at night gives them a restful sleep and doesn't induce the awake feeling that can happen during the day.

These conflicting studies or anecdotes may have to do with the fact that CBD has what's called a bidirectional or biphasic effect related to the endocannabinoid system. That means depending on the dosage, CBD might either improve sleep or induce wakefulness. In moderate doses, CBD can act as a stimulant, like caffeine, according to Project CBD.

Depending on why you have insomnia can also make a difference in how CBD oil affects you. One case study, for example, showed that a young girl with post-traumatic stress disorder used CBD oil to help her sleep better and reduce anxiety.

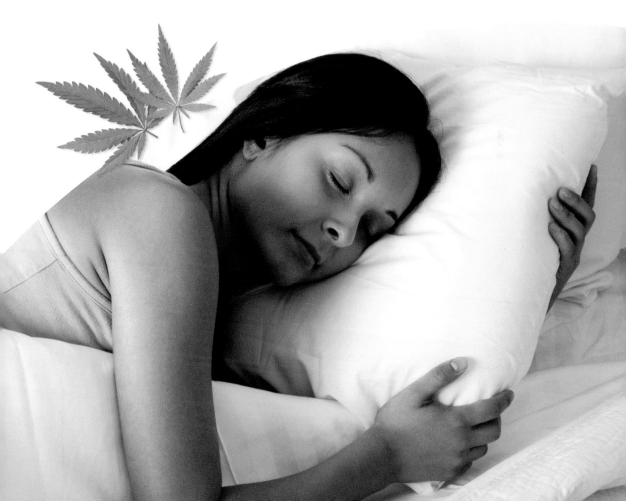

# Menopause and PMS

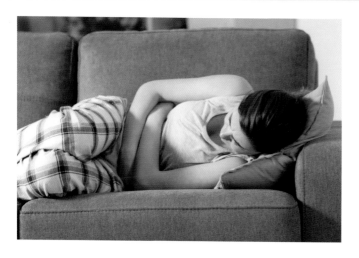

Women experience various symptoms when having their monthly period. Some can be mild; others can be severe. Premenstrual syndrome typically occurs a week or so before menstruation. Symptoms include bloating, depression, headache, irritability, fatigue, acne, abdominal cramps, and mood swings. Roughly eighty-five percent of women experience at least one PMS symptom monthly, according to the American College of Obstetricians and Gynecologists.

If these are severe, a woman may be diagnosed with premenstrual dysphoric disorder (PMDD). Hormonal changes likely contribute to PMS and PMDD. Depression and major stress can trigger these disorders. Serotonin levels drop when a woman suffers from PMS, and that could relate to depression, which is also characterized by low serotonin levels.

Over-the-counter medications can treat pain and cramping. Taking calcium, vitamin D, and magnesium may also help.

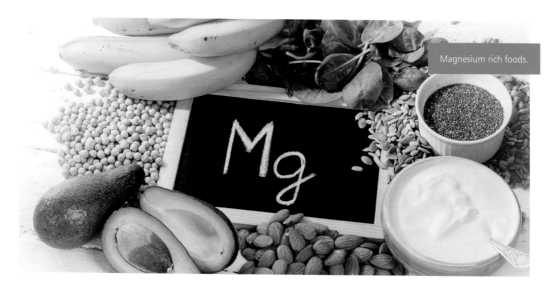

Magnesium rich foods.

# PMS and CBD

Dr. Judy Holland, a psychiatrist who has written books on women's issues, believes CBD could help with PMS because of its anti-inflammatory properties. She also thinks it might be able to relieve anxiety and relax the uterine muscles where cramping occurs. CBD tinctures have been recommended to ease PMS symptoms.

# Menopause Symptoms

Before a woman reaches menopause, she may experience some symptoms and signs including irregular periods, hot flashes, chills, night sweats, mood changes, and weight gain. Menopause occurs when a woman's reproductive hormones decline, and eventually the ovaries stop producing eggs. Menopause, a natural biological change, typically occurs when a woman is in her forties or fifties.

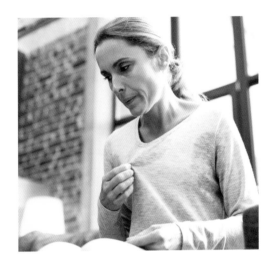

Menopause begins when a woman has not menstruated for at least a year, and hot flashes and night sweats, among other symptoms, can occur for several years after the onset of menopause.

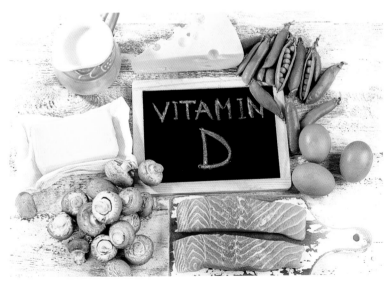

No treatment is necessary for women undergoing menopause, but sometimes the symptoms are so bothersome that certain medications are prescribed. Hot flashes can be relieved with hormone therapy, which can help prevent bone loss, but in the long term may cause some cardiovascular issues, and has been linked to breast cancer. Some physicians prescribe antidepressants in low dosages to help women who cannot take hormone therapy or who suffer from mood changes during menopause. Physicians also recommend vitamin D to keep bones strong and reduce the risk of fractures.

Avoiding caffeine, not smoking, and exercising regularly are also considered ways to cope with bothersome symptoms of menopause. Black cohosh has been recommended as an alternative treatment, but the Mayo Clinic says it's not helpful and could be harmful.

# Menopause and CBD

One study showed that CBD could help curb bone density loss, which occurs during and after menopause, but few other studies have been done on this issue. Women undergoing menopause have anecdotally reported that taking CBD either via an oil or by a vape pen has helped reduce their symptoms. CBD has been said to block the production of a chemical that breaks down a natural cannabinoid in the body that regulates body temperature. It's possible that's why using CBD might be able to lessen hot flashes. One study also suggested CBD could relieve insomnia related to menopause.

Some researchers believe that lower estrogen levels in a woman's body during menopause might disrupt the human endocannabinoid system that regulates mood—and that could be what causes anxiety and depression during menopause.

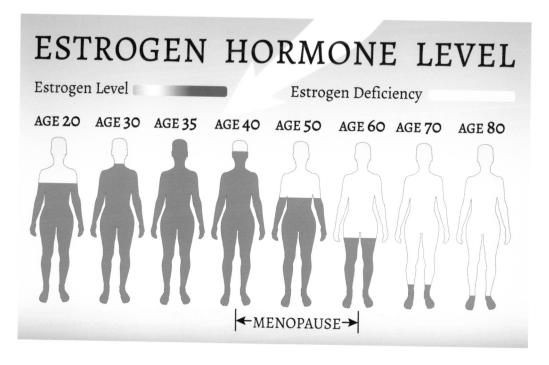

# Migraines

Headaches, one of the most common health issues, range from annoying to debilitating. A wide variety of headaches exist and come from various causes, especially stress and tension, as well as hangovers, and some diseases such as glaucoma, even a poor diet. A physician can help determine if it's a migraine.

Most headaches are tension headaches, which usually affect the whole head, and can feel like a band is wrapped around the skull. They can also affect the muscles of the neck and shoulders, causing aching and stiffness. The pain is usually mild to moderate—although it can occasionally be severe. Headache pain normally lasts a few hours and is typically a chronic, steady pain.

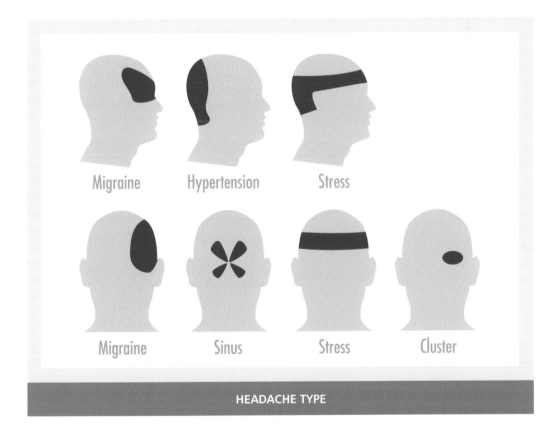

Migraine   Hypertension   Stress

Migraine   Sinus   Stress   Cluster

**HEADACHE TYPE**

A migraine usually affects one side of the head, is moderately to severely painful, and has a throbbing quality that can be worsened by exertion. Migraines also are often accompanied by other symptoms called auras, which can include nausea or vomiting; sensitivity to light, sound, or smells; vision changes; and numbness. Aura symptoms can occur ten to thirty minutes before the

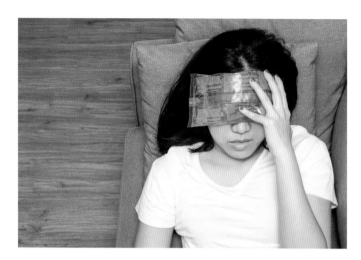

migraine occurs. Some sufferers also experience subtle symptoms a day or two before getting a migraine, such as constipation, depression, irritability, or unusual mood changes. In addition, patients can suffer from what are called ocular migraines, which don't necessarily cause headaches, but cause temporary light spots in one or both eyes. They're temporary, usually about a half hour long and likely not dangerous, though any eye disturbance should be reported to a physician.

Migraines typically last from four to seventy hours or even longer. Though the reasons for getting migraines aren't known, they are likely caused by cervical spine issues or problems with the brain's blood and nerve vessels.

Migraines affect thirty-eight million Americans and are considered one of the world's most disabling illnesses. Those who have chronic migraines also suffer from depression, anxiety, and sleep disorders.

# Migraine Treatment

Like tension headaches, migraines are first treated with over-the-counter medications like acetaminophen, aspirin, and ibuprofen. Some over-the-counter medications specifically marketed for migraines combine one or more of these drugs with caffeine, which helps the medication work more quickly. But when these remedies don't work, prescription drugs may be used to help the blood vessels around the brain contract and to increase serotonin levels in the brain. Anti-nausea drugs may also be prescribed. But when none of these options work, doctors may prescribe opioids like codeine or oxycodone.

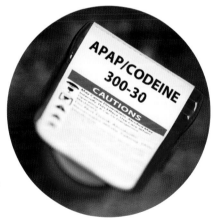

Stress management also can work; and recently, Botox, which most recognize as a cosmetic treatment to reduce wrinkles, has also been used to treat people with migraines and muscular issues.

# Migraines and CBD

Some studies indicate a deficiency in the endocannabinoid system might cause migraine headaches, and it's thought that using CBD might be able to fix the deficiency. Some physicians treat migraine patients with CBD oil, but no studies pointing to its efficacy exist. Some anecdotal evidence comes from patients, for example, a man who suffered from both ocular and painful migraines found CBD therapy to eliminate the symptoms.

One physician has recommended CBD capsule for those who suffer with anxiety and tight muscles in the cervix—those symptoms, for some, were alleviated with the capsule, but there could be no correlation between CBD and migraines.

An important concept to note is that sometimes some medicines can help headaches as well as cause them—and that may be true for CBD. One of the most commonly reported side effects of CBD includes headache—but that may have to do with dosages, product quality, and other issues. Some migraine sufferers say CBD helps; but others don't.

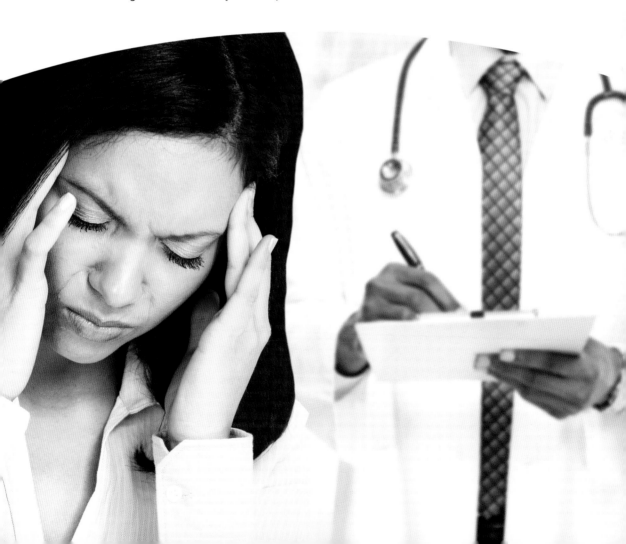

# Multiple Sclerosis

"Sclerosis" refers to a hardening of tissue. In the case of multiple sclerosis, the tissue affected is the substance that surrounds and protects nerve fibers, called myelin. In this disease, the immune system causes inflammation that damages or destroys myelin, leaving behind scar tissue in multiple areas. When this happens, messages within the central nervous system are altered or even stopped, resulting in a variety of neurological symptoms.

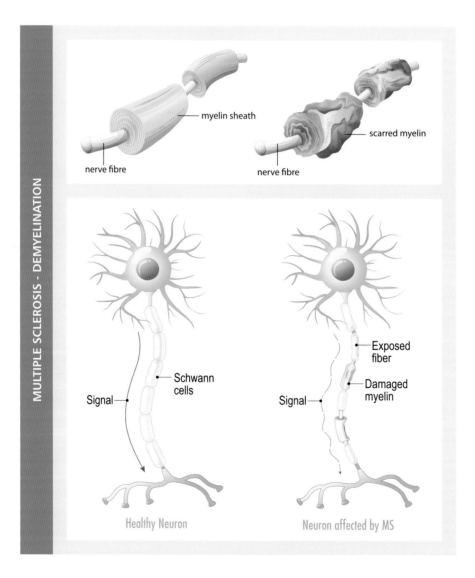

MULTIPLE SCLEROSIS - DEMYELINATION

myelin sheath

scarred myelin

nerve fibre

nerve fibre

Exposed fiber

Schwann cells

Damaged myelin

Signal

Signal

Healthy Neuron

Neuron affected by MS

A combination of environmental and genetic conditions can contribute to the development of MS, although the actual cause is not known. Strangely, the rate of MS is more common among people who live farther away from the equator than people who live closer to the equator. Also, some experts debate whether microbes and infectious agents cause MS to develop.

# MS Symptoms

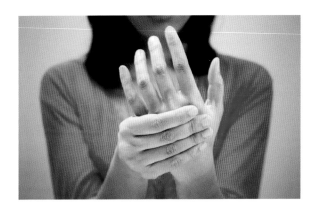

Symptoms of the disease vary from person to person and can be random and unpredictable, making it difficult at times to definitively diagnose the disorder. But some of the most common symptoms include fatigue, weakness, numbness or tingling in the face, body, or extremities, walking difficulties, muscle spasms, dizziness, and vision problems. Depression is also an extremely common symptom—in fact, depression is more common in MS patients than in the general population or among those with other chronic conditions.

Less common symptoms can include speech problems, tremors, difficulty swallowing, breathing problems, and seizures. Secondary symptoms can also arise as a result of the primary symptoms of the disease; for instance, a difficulty with walking can result in weakened muscles or a loss of bone density. MS sufferers may also eventually be unable to continue working, or feel that dealing with their disease leaves them isolated from family and friends.

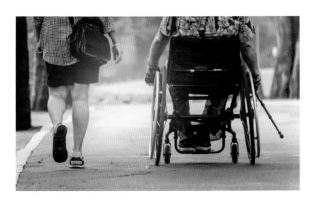

An astonishing amount of symptoms are associated with recognizing and diagnosing multiple sclerosis. Any number of neurological signs occur during the disease's onset, with automatic, visual, motor, and sensory problems topping the list. Sufferers of MS may feel a lack of or change in sensory perception, tingling, numbness, muscle spasms, weakness, and blurred vision.

The disease generally begins with a single first episode, known as clinically isolated syndrome, which is characteristic of MS, but does not always develop into the disease. If another episode occurs, an official diagnosis of MS may be made. Most patients—about eighty-five percent—are afflicted with relapse-remitting MS, which consists of periods of symptom-free remissions interspersed with episodes of new or worsening symptoms. But eventually, the disease can progress to the point of fewer remissions and a steady deterioration of symptoms.

# MS Treatments

MS has no cure, so treatments aim to control symptoms. The most commonly prescribed drugs are corticosteroids, which reduce inflammation and suppress the immune system to prevent it from attacking healthy tissue. A number of drugs can also be prescribed to slow the progression of the disease, and these can either be injected, taken in pill form, or administered by intravenous infusion. Physical therapy is often used to help patients restore coordination and strengthen muscles.

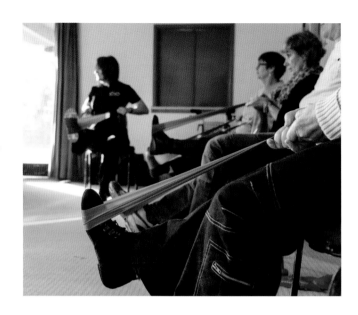

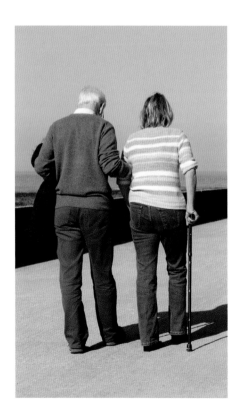

# MS and CBD

One woman tried opioids prescribed by her physician to deal with pain and depression symptoms from her MS. When that didn't work, he suggested medical marijuana, but she did not like the psychoactive effects. She then tried using CBD and discovered she was able to find relief without getting high.

In Canada, CBD has been used as a supplemental treatment for spasticity, one of the common symptoms of MS. Spasticity refers to a condition in which some muscles continuously contract causing stiffness and tightness and interfering with normal movement and speech. Few studies have been done on the effects of CBD oil on MS patients, and experts say while CBD oil cannot cure MS, it might be able to provide relief from bothersome symptoms.

# Pain and Opioid Abuse

Pain may be the most basic and ubiquitous malady affecting humans. We've all felt it—everything from a tiny splinter under the skin to a broken bone can cause unpleasant, or even unbearable, sensations. Pain can be sharp, burning, dull, or achy; the pain we feel from a headache is different from the pain we feel from a sunburn. If the onset is sudden and lasts only a short amount of time, it is acute pain; but if it is unrelenting and lasts for months—or longer—it is chronic pain.

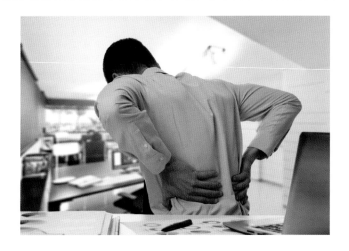

As upsetting as pain is, it has an important function: mainly, to alert you of a dangerous situation within your body. The nerve cells that produce pain are part of the peripheral nervous system, which includes all of the body's nerves except those in the spine and brain, which make up the central nervous system. When nerve endings are stimulated—such as when you stub your toe or cut yourself—special peripheral nerve cells called nociceptors send a pain message in the form of electrical impulses to the brain.

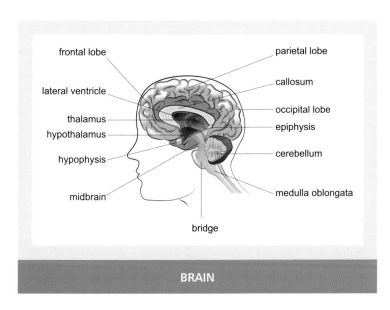

frontal lobe

parietal lobe

lateral ventricle

callosum

occipital lobe

thalamus

epiphysis

hypothalamus

hypophysis

cerebellum

midbrain

medulla oblongata

bridge

**BRAIN**

Painful stimulus in the hand, for example, sends information through nerves that travel up the pathways along the spinal column and up to the thalamus. The thalamus consists of two different masses of gray matter that are positioned between the two cerebral hemispheres. The thalamus is responsible for pain perception and relaying sensory information.

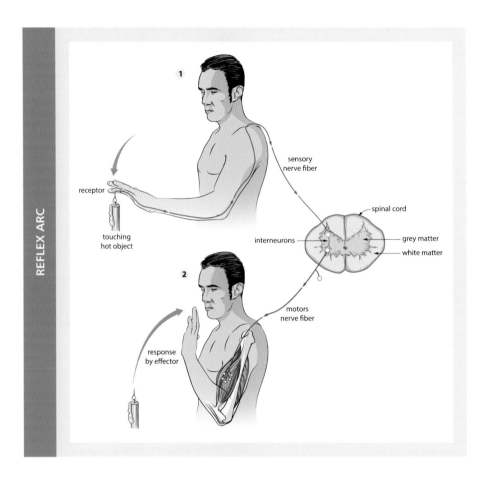

The International Association for the Study of Pain originally classified pain with five criteria: 1) where on the body it occurs, 2) anatomical system causing the pain, 3) duration and pattern of pain, 4) intensity, and 5) cause. However, this type of classification has come under some scrutiny from Harvard Medical School neurobiologist Clifford J. Woolf, who has created a new set of criteria for understanding pain. These criteria are 1) nociceptive pain, which is caused by stimulation of the sensory nerve fibers, 2) inflammatory pain associated with tissue and immune cell damages, and 3) pathological pain, which is caused by damage to the nervous system.

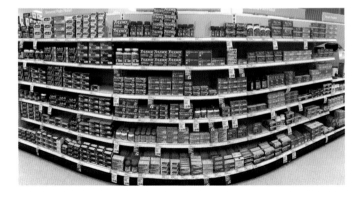

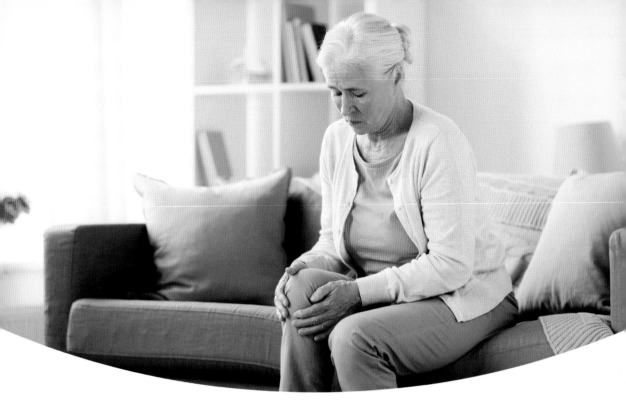

# Perceiving Pain

How you ultimately perceive pain depends on several factors. Genetics play a role, not only with pain tolerance but also with how you respond to pain medications. Psychological factors can come into play as well—those who suffer from depression and anxiety tend to feel more pain than those who don't. Even having a pessimistic attitude toward pain can make it feel worse. Past experiences can also influence how pain is perceived: If you've already had a painful past experience with a situation—for example, at the dentist—your body is more likely to produce a pain response during subsequent scenarios. Interestingly, the biggest risk factor for developing a painful condition is having already experienced a painful condition.

The spinal cord actually sorts through the messages from these nociceptors to determine their urgency. Burning pain from a hot stove is deemed urgent, which then triggers your muscles to react by moving away from the source of the heat. But the pain from a mild scratch is relayed more slowly, resulting merely in a bit of discomfort. Once the pain messages reach the brain, the brain can send out its own messages, like signaling white blood cells to rush to an injury site, or flooding the body with pain-suppressing endorphins.

Pain from a scratch is relayed more slowly than pain from a burn.

# Pain Treatment

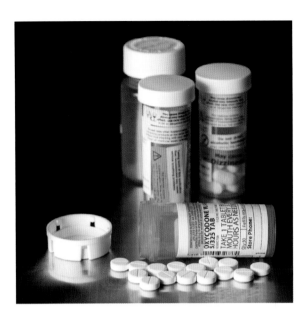

It's obvious that pain is a complex process, and certainly one we'd all prefer to avoid. So when patients are overwhelmed with unrelenting pain, they're grateful to try any treatments their doctors may offer. Many times, that treatment plan includes opioid pain medications such as hydrocodone, fentanyl, and morphine. These narcotics work by binding to receptors in the brain and blocking all those pain messages sent by the peripheral nervous system. They're sort of like bouncers standing outside a nightclub—pain may be all dressed up, but because an opioid is standing in front of the velvet rope, it has nowhere to go.

Opioids can be very effective at managing chronic pain, but they come with some serious drawbacks. They can be highly addictive, especially when needed for long-term pain. And once use is discontinued, they can cause uncomfortable withdrawal symptoms like insomnia, vomiting, muscle and bone pain, and chills. But even worse than addiction and withdrawal is the possibility of overdose: When taken in large doses, or combined with other medications or alcohol, opioids can cause users to stop breathing. And frighteningly, this scenario plays out nearly 175 times a day in the United States.

# Pain and CBD

Medical marijuana with high THC content has been used to lessen pain. In one study, almost three thousand patients who used opioids and cannabis to control their pain were surveyed. Of those patients, ninety-seven percent reported that cannabis allowed them to decrease their opioid use. And eighty-one percent said that cannabis alone was even more effective than cannabis combined with opioids.

But what about using CBD, which can be obtained over the counter or online and which doesn't produce the psychoactive effect? First, CBD has been shown to decrease inflammation, which relates to reducing pain. An animal study indicated that CBD could be used to lessen chronic pain.

A small study suggested that the CBD helps to reduce cravings of heroin addicts, which might be useful to those wanting to break their addictions to opioids.

In addition, a drug called Sativex, not approved in the U.S., has been used in Europe and Canada to treat pain that opioids cannot help. The drug has a one to one CBD to THC ratio. The FDA is considering approving Sativex for cancer patients with pain.

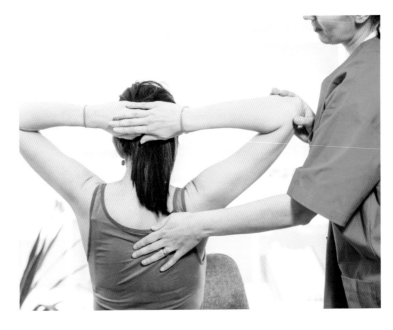

Studies are now being done to see how chronic pain sufferers react when put on a regimen of high CBD and low THC treatment.

Anecdotal evidence suggests CBD may be able to lessen pain. A Colorado-based man who suffered muscle and joint pain related to sports injuries tried prescription medication to treat the pain. He later decided to try a topical CBD. He found that back pain he got when hiking could be subdued by using the topical CBD.

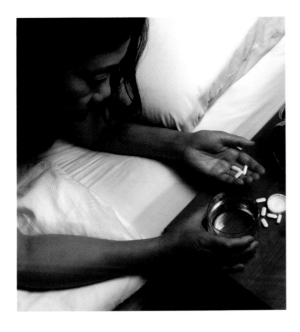

# Opioid Addiction, Overdoses and CBD

Reducing opioid overdoses is one benefit of treating pain with CBD. Opioids can cause cognitive impairment, to the point that those who are using them for severe pain may not even be able to communicate and function.

More than 11 million people misuse prescription opioids, according to the U.S. Department of Health and Human Services. More than 49,000 people died from opioid abuse, including overdose, in 2016, according to the National Institute on Drug Abuse.

Recent studies on both animals and humans show that CBD may be able to help with drug addiction, including opioids. A physician and director of an addiction institute in Mount Sinai has done research on the brain activity of opioid addicts. She said opioids damage certain receptors in the brain, which cause humans to make poor decisions and continue taking opioids. She thinks that CBD normalizes the receptors and helps reduce cravings, and some believe that means CBD oil could be effective in treating addiction.

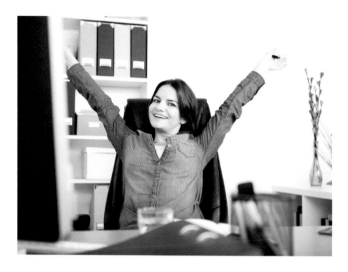

Though its use in treating addiction is not approved by the FDA, some football players in the National Football League who have abused opioids reportedly switched to using CBD for their pain relief. The NFL does not approve the usage of CBD for pain relief by football players.

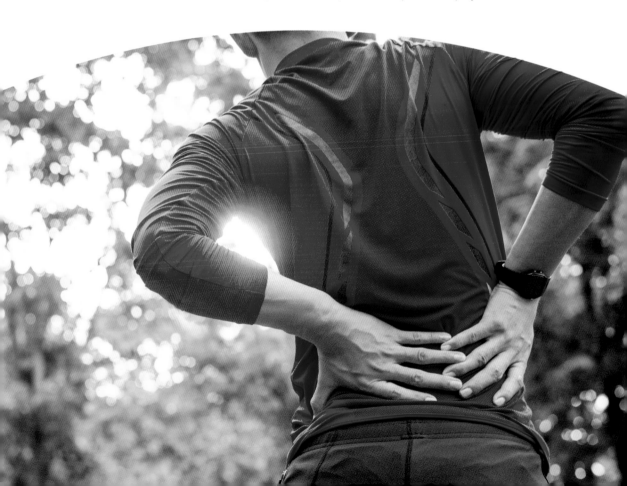

# Parkinson's Disease

Parkinson's disease—an incurable and progressive brain disorder—affects about one million people in the United States. People with this disease experience a wide range of differing symptoms; no two people with Parkinson's are alike. But all of those who suffer from this disease have one thing in common: A loss of dopamine-producing neurons in an area of the brain that is responsible for body movement and coordination. And it is not until a substantial number of these neurons die—about eighty percent—that symptoms begin to appear.

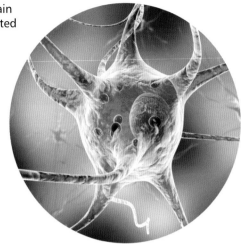

## Parkinson's Symptoms

Symptoms of Parkinson's usually begin slowly—early signs of the disease can be so mild that they go unnoticed. Sometimes the only indication that something is amiss is a slight tremor in one hand or a feeling of stiffness. Other symptoms include slowed movement, rigid muscles, impaired balance, or speech or writing changes. Some people also notice difficulty performing unconscious movements like swinging their arms when they walk.

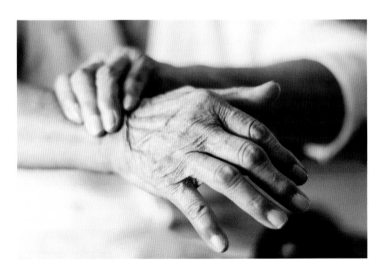

Often the preliminary symptoms will begin on only one side of the body, but as the disease progresses, both sides of the body can be affected. Tremors and coordination become increasingly worse, and activities like walking, eating, and dressing can be difficult. Eventually, a walker or wheelchair may be needed, and those in the late stages of the disease often need round-the-clock care to function.

Most of those with Parkinson's disease first show symptoms after the age of fifty; but between two and ten percent of those with the disease are under the age of fifty. One of these patients—the actor Michael J. Fox—was only twenty-nine years old when he was diagnosed.

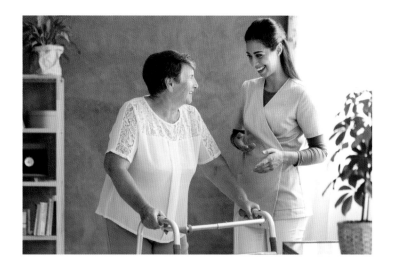

# Parkinson's Treatments

Treatments include prescription medications to replenish dopamine, which may temporarily reduce tremors and improve coordination, or other drugs that help to suppress the effects of the disease. If medications don't work, surgery may be an option. Implantable devices called deep brain stimulators can send electrical impulses to the area of the brain that is malfunctioning, stopping tremors and improving coordination. Other treatments include healthy lifestyle changes like adding in regular exercise, and eating a diet that includes plenty of vitamins C, D, and E.

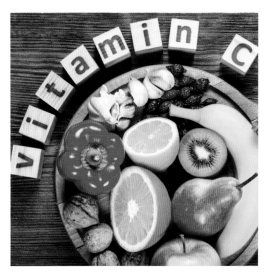

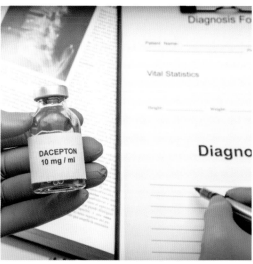

Aside from turning toward surgery or medications to treat Parkinson's, patients can use other methods to maintain mobility and manage pain. According to the magazine *Parkinson's Disease*, there is scarce evidence that rehabilitation practices can improve mobility and speech difficulties. But patients under the care of a physiotherapist tend to manage better, and even exercise not supervised under the umbrella of physical rehabilitation can help patients remain mobile, flexible, and strong. The Lee Silverman voice treatment approach to treating speech impairments is widely practiced to help patients with their declining speech functions.

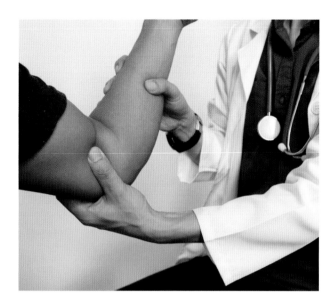

# Parkinson's and CBD

For decades—centuries, even—people with Parkinson's have been praising cannabis for its ability to reduce tremors. Some studies have found that the neuroprotective properties of cannabis may help prevent brain cells from dying and prevent the buildup of neurotoxins which contribute to the disease.

One 2014 study showed Parkinson's patients improved their sense of well-being and quality of life after being treated with CBD. One study showed that 300 mg of CBD improved the quality of life and that 150 mg of CBD over four weeks reduced psychotic symptoms, while an oral dosage of CBD from 75–300 mg improved sleep disorders resulting from the disease.

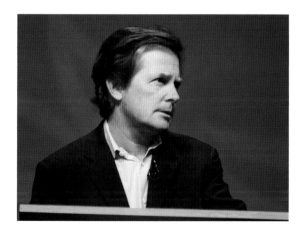

Michael J. Fox, who has used marijuana to treat his disease, is also a proponent of CBD oil, because it doesn't contain enough THC to cause psychoactive effects. A strain of CBD oil that contains some THC is considered to be helpful in controlling pain, muscle spasms, and side effects of other medications. Getting the correct ratio of THC to CBD could reduce symptoms more easily, researchers are discovering. Many more clinical trials are needed to see how CBD oil affects Parkinson's patients.

# Post-Traumatic Stress Disorder

When we think of post-traumatic stress disorder, or PTSD, we often think of soldiers returning from war. And this is definitely a risk factor: Up to thirty percent of military personnel who have served in wars suffer from the disorder. But PTSD can affect anyone who has experienced frightening, life-threatening, or traumatic events, such as natural disasters, serious accidents, terrorist attacks, or sexual assault. It is estimated that about eight percent of Americans—around 24 million people—have PTSD, and seventy percent of Americans will experience at least one traumatic event during their lives.

Those who suffer from the disorder may have nightmares or flashbacks of their frightening experience, or may relive the trauma when confronted with reminders of the incident. These symptoms can cause them to avoid certain people, places, or activities that might trigger unwanted memories. Sufferers can develop depression, memory problems, personality changes, and issues with substance abuse—more than half of all men with PTSD have problems with alcohol. Eventually, they might lose their ability to function in normal social situations. Job loss, divorce, relationship issues, and parenting problems are all common. Traumatic events can cause our bodies to over-respond by releasing too much adrenaline, creating deeply embedded neurological patterns

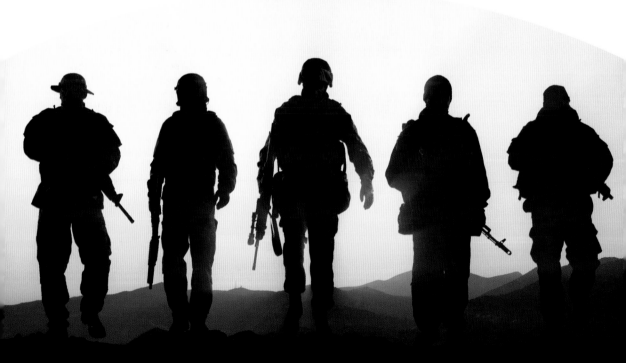

that can make the person fearful of traumatic events in the future. Soldiers are constantly exposed to traumatic events of all sorts, including the detonation of artillery.

Post-traumatic stress disorder is associated with several regions of the brain. Patients of PTSD often have less brain function in their prefrontal cortex, which is responsible for experiencing and controlling emotions.

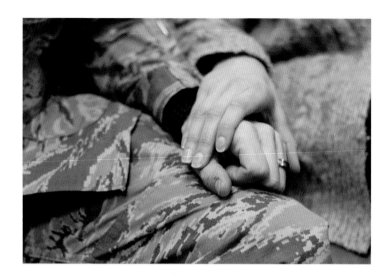

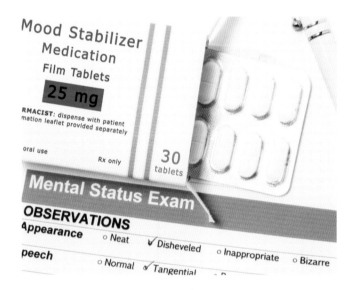

## PTSD Treatment

The main treatments for PTSD include therapy and medications like antidepressants or sleeping pills. Therapy aims to help people face and control their fears, as well as learn relaxation and anger management skills. As a last resort, antipsychotic drugs may be prescribed. The side effects, unfortunately, can be serious and can include weight gain, elevated cholesterol levels, muscle rigidity, and involuntary tremors, which may become permanent.

# PTSD and CBD

People suffering from PTSD have been found to have an endocannabinoid deficiency. CBD in marijuana has been shown to help PTSD sufferers desensitize to triggers that remind them of their past experience. However, some experts say veterans with PTSD could develop dependence on marijuana, which has a high THC content.

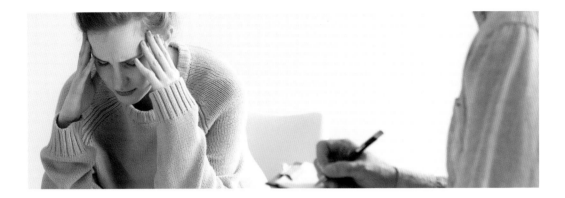

Using CBD, which doesn't produce psychoactive effects, might be able to treat PTSD symptoms based on various studies. For example, CBD has also been shown to disrupt the recollection of long-term memories, helping them fade into the background. Another study done with rats suggests that CBD can help treat PTSD by alleviating some of its long-lasting effects.

A case study presented in a paper about PTSD and CBD showed a 10-year-old girl suffering from PTSD due to sexual abuse and other issues. She took prescribed medications but relief only lasted for a while, and side effects became an issue.

She was put on a CBD oil regimen that helped control her anxiety and improve her sleep. The study's authors said the case study shows CBD oil can be effective in reduce anxiety and insomnia associated with PTSD, especially in the light of the fact that the patient received no other pharmaceutical medications besides CBD.

Another anecdote showed that an army veteran who also experienced sexual abuse found CBD reduces anxiety, which improved sleep. A person from Pennsylvania also stated that treating PTSD with CBD enabled the patient to stop taking all but one antidepressant.

Some animal studies also suggest that CBD may work with the brain during REM or rapid eye movement during sleep.

In treating PTSD, researchers are also considering various strains of cannabinoids, which could contain different ratios of THC and CBD.

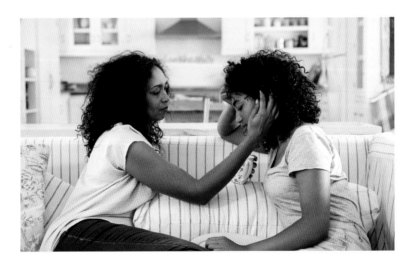

# Schizophrenia

Schizophrenia is a chronic, often debilitating, mental disease that cannot be cured, but only managed with various treatments. Those with schizophrenia behave as if they are not in touch with reality.

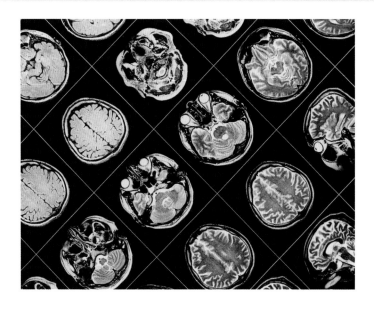

More than 2 million Americans have schizophrenic episodes annually, and one in five could completely recover. Symptoms of this biological illness typically begin when a person is between the ages of sixteen and thirty, and can become worse, then better, then worse again.

Causes include genetics, brain chemistry, and certain types of drug use, as well as exposures to certain viruses.

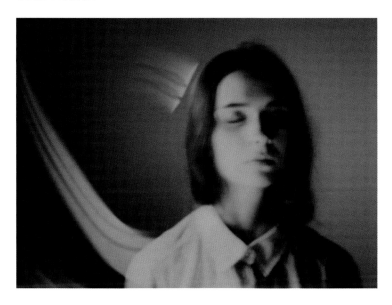

Symptoms are placed into three types. One type is called positive, in which a patient has hallucinations, uncontrollable movement, and delusions. Another type called negative involves difficulties in maintaining speech, starting and ending projects, and enjoying life. The third type, cognitive, includes symptoms of lost memory, difficulty focusing, and inability to think clearly. Cognitive symptoms can be mild to severe.

# Treatment

Psychiatrists typically treat those suffering with schizophrenia by prescribing anti-psychotic medicines. Some of these have side effects, and a physician works with a patient to find the best drug with the least side effects. Those with schizophrenia also work with trained psychologists who can help them cope with their symptoms and 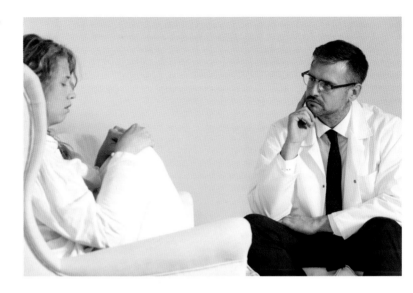 lead a quality life. According to the National Institute of Mental Health those who regularly work on what are called psychosocial treatments are less likely to be hospitalized from the disease or have serious relapses.

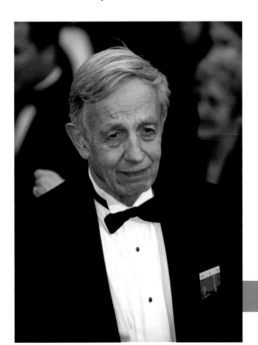

John Nash at the Academy Awards

Those with the disease can also find relief through combining all the treatments mentioned above, as well as getting their families involved and joining support groups.

Many have likely seen the movie *A Beautiful Mind*, based on a true story about a mathematical genius named John Nash who battled with schizophrenia for many decades. Disliking the side effects from his medication, he stopped taking them and declared that he had willed himself to combat his symptoms without any medication. Some physicians say Nash's diagnosis of schizophrenia may not have been correct, and do not believe those with true schizophrenia can will themselves out of the disease.

# Schizophrenia and CBD

Products with high THC content, i.e., marijuana, have been said to exacerbate the psychotic symptoms of those with the disease and increase their anxiety. Some studies negate the belief that smoking marijuana can worsen schizophrenia, leaving open the path to the potential for CBD, which doesn't have the psychoactive effects of marijuana, to treat the disease.

One study showed CBD has antipsychotic effects similar to the drugs prescribed to schizophrenics. Nineteen patients received an antipsychotic drug; another twenty received CBD and each found similar relief. However, side effects associated with the antipsychotics weren't seen in the patients who took CBD.

One chemical that changes within the brain of someone with schizophrenia is called dopamine, which processes pleasure, movement, and emotions. Scientists think low dopamine levels may be related to psychotic episodes experienced by those with schizophrenia. Some studies suggest CBD oil may increase the activity of dopamine in the brain.

Another study pointed to the fact that one-third of schizophrenic patients don't receive good relief from their symptoms with antipsychotic drugs, which is why more research needs to be done on how CBD may be able to help. The study suggested that CBD might be able to improve the effects of antipsychotic drugs as well as reduce stress and inflammation associated with the disease. One study, however, showed that CBD used alone without any other treatment may not have the same therapeutic effects on those with schizophrenia.

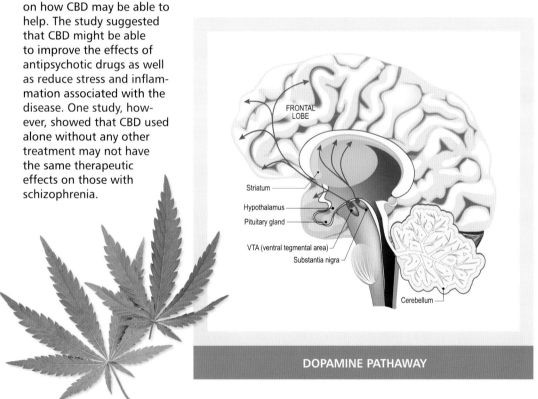

Striatum

Hypothalamus

Pituitary gland

VTA (ventral tegmental area)

Substantia nigra

FRONTAL LOBE

Cerebellum

**DOPAMINE PATHAWAY**

# Skin Conditions and Disorders

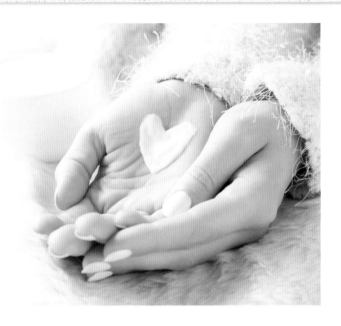

The largest organ in our bodies is the skin. It serves us well by absorbing oxygen as well as nutrients such as Vitamin D. It's also water resistant, and when the endocannabinoid system is in balance, the skin should be free of itching, dryness, and other issues. Cannabinoid receptors are found through the cells in our skin—and that's why some recommend using topical solutions with CBD to help with acne and other problems.

Hormonal imbalances, diet, disrupted immune system, and allergies can all cause skin problems.

## Dry, Itchy Skin, Rashes, and Bug Bites

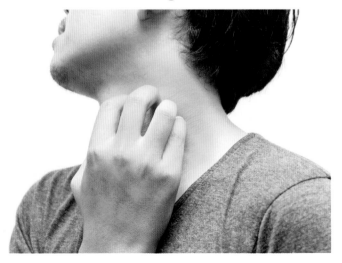

Our skin is deluged by a host of enemies including cold, windy weather, insect bites, heat, and overexposure to allergies and the sun, as well as a stressed immune system. These can cause dry, itchy skin, rashes, sores, burns, and discoloration. And, of course, in the case of sunburn, there's the possibility of skin cancer.

Various creams, sprays, and other products are prescribed to help reduce these symptoms. If inflammation is causing the problem, CBD is said

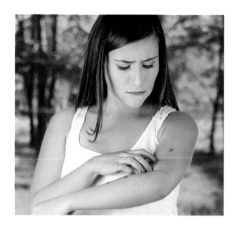

to be able to help because of its anti-inflammatory properties. Some CBD products contain fatty acids that help keep skin moisturized. A study done in a dermatology department at a university school of medicine showed that eight out of twenty-one patients who used topical CBD creams twice a day for three weeks no longer had severely itchy skin. Another study showed that topical creams with high amounts of CBD helped reduce itching problems. In addition, CBD is an anti-inflammatory, according to some researchers, meaning it may help rashes caused by inflammation. CBD is said to have anti-bacterial properties, which could help when used on bug bites.

# Acne and CBD

Acne is a very common skin condition that not only plagues teenagers, but also adults. Stress can cause acne in people of all ages. It's basically a reaction to clogged pores in the skin. Over-the-counter and prescription medications are used to help those with acne. But some of these products can damage sensitive skin and create other issues. CBD applied topically is said to reduce inflammation caused by acne as well as prevent damage such as scarring. One study showed that CBD can slow the production of lipids, which could prevent acne from intensifying.

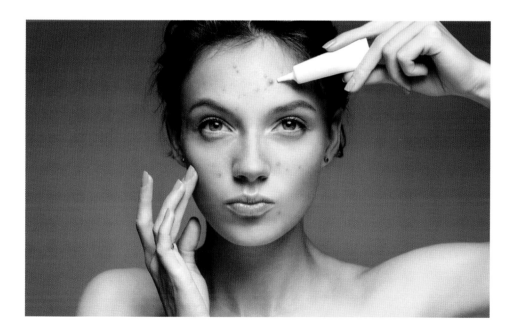

# Psoriasis

Psoriasis is an autoimmune and genetic disease triggered by environmental factors such as infections, medications, trauma, stress, and cold. Psoriasis also has been said to increase the risk of getting psoriatic arthritis, Crohn's disease, depression, and heart disease. At least 7.5 million Americans suffer from psoriasis.

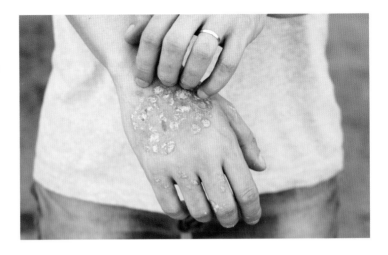

No cure is available for the inflammatory condition, which causes skin cells to mature too rapidly, which in turn leads to skin tissue ulcerations and pain.

Physicians perform a physical exam to determine if someone has psoriasis. Occasionally, physicians take a small skin sample to rule out other issues.

# Conventional and Alternative Treatments

Topical creams and prescription drugs are used to treat psoriasis, though some of them may be costly or have unwanted side effects. Other treatments involve using artificial ultraviolet light.

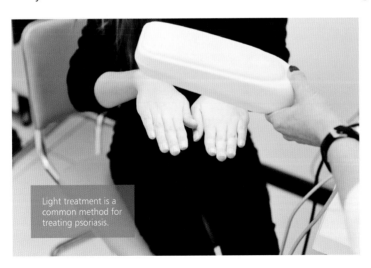

Light treatment is a common method for treating psoriasis.

In some cases, the light treatments greatly reduce the symptoms. Sunlight exposure may also help, but the problem is that sunlight exposure also can cause skin cancer.

Some patients may benefit from acupuncture as well as dietary changes, meditation, and relaxation techniques, according to the National Psoriasis Foundation.

# Psoriasis and CBD

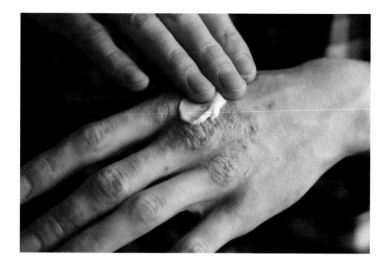

With psoriasis, skin cells, which typically are replenished every thirty days, may be replaced in as little as three days, causing inflammation. Research has shown that CBD may be able to protect against inflammation as well as the buildup of dead skin which occurs in psoriasis patients. Another study showed CBD could help those with arthritis, which is one disorder that can develop in psoriasis patients.

# Eczema

More than 30 million Americans suffer from some type of eczema, a condition characterized by inflamed, red, and itchy skin as well as dark or leathery patches on the skin, and swelling. Physicians can diagnose specific types of eczema through skin examinations and other methods.

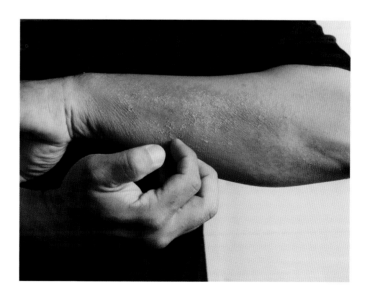

The most common form of eczema is called atopic dermatitis, and knowing the root cause, for example, if it's related to some sort of auto-immune disease, could help reduce flare ups and reduce symptoms.

The word eczema comes from Greek words meaning "to boil over," because in more severe cases, the skin can get blisters and peel.

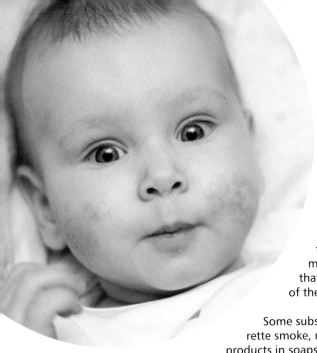

Babies and children often develop eczema on their cheeks, but it can happen anywhere on the body. For some children, it goes away; for others, it remains through their adult years. In addition, adults who never had eczema as a child can develop the condition.

Researchers don't know specifically what causes eczema, but believe it involves genetics, an autoimmune deficiency, and some sort of trigger by a substance within or outside the body. Some eczema patients also have a mutation of a gene that creates a type of protein that maintains a protective barrier on the top layer of the skin.

Some substances that might trigger eczema include cigarette smoke, nickel, perfumes, and formaldehyde, as well as products in soaps, cleaners, shampoos, and lotions. Stress can also cause flare ups in those with eczema. No cure is available, but many treatments exist.

# Treatment

As with psoriasis, treatment can involve over-the-counter or prescribed medications that are either used topically, orally, or via injection. Moisturizers are also recommended. Some natural treatments include taking a bath with oatmeal or baking soda or creating a paste and applying it to the skin. Apple cider vinegar baths have also been recommended. Using bath oils can help, too, as long as they don't contain any irritants or allergens that would further trigger the eczema instead of calming it.

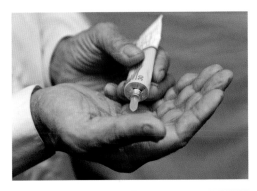

As with psoriasis, light therapy has also been used to treat eczema. In severe cases, some patients have been prescribed a type of antidepressant that can relieve itching at night.

Another natural method designed to calm the skin and enhance the use of topical creams is called wet wrap therapy. The technique involves dampening certain cotton materials with warm

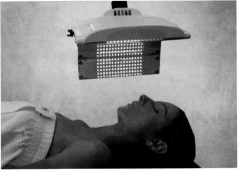

water and then wrapping it around the skin where the eczema is occurring. A dry layer is then wrapped around the wet one. Leaving wet wraps on for at least several hours is recommended.

# Eczema and CBD

Anecdotal evidence has shown that CBD could help some eczema patients. One woman from Great Britain had suffered with mild eczema, which became severe after she became pregnant. It did not clear up after her daughter was born. She tried steroids, itching cream, and light therapy to no avail. After being hospitalized for the disorder, she tried vaping CBD, and her skin cleared in about two weeks.

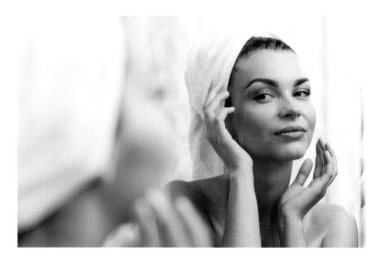

One study showed applying CBD topically could ease the itchiness and inflammation caused by eczema, as well as other skin conditions. Topical CBD may be helpful in treating various skin conditions including psoriasis and eczema, according to a study published by the *Journal of the American Academy of Dermatology*.

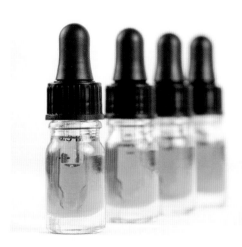

Choosing the right CBD product is important for those with eczema because extra ingredients could irritate the condition. Some CBD creams contain what are called terpenes, which can be helpful with some disorders, but are said to make conditions worse for those with eczema.

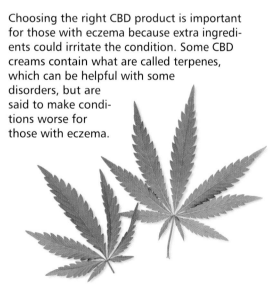

# Smoking Cessation

Most people understand that smoking tobacco is harmful to the health. It's been linked to lung cancer, heart disease, respiratory diseases, and premature death. The drug, nicotine, found in tobacco, can also cause an addiction in most smokers. That makes it difficult for people to stop —indeed, some research indicates nicotine can be as addictive as cocaine or alcohol. Cigarette smoking is the leading cause of preventable disease and death in the United States, accounting for more than 480,000 deaths every year, or about one in five deaths, according to the Centers for Disease Control and Prevention. More than 41,000 of these deaths are related to secondhand smoke, according to the CDC.

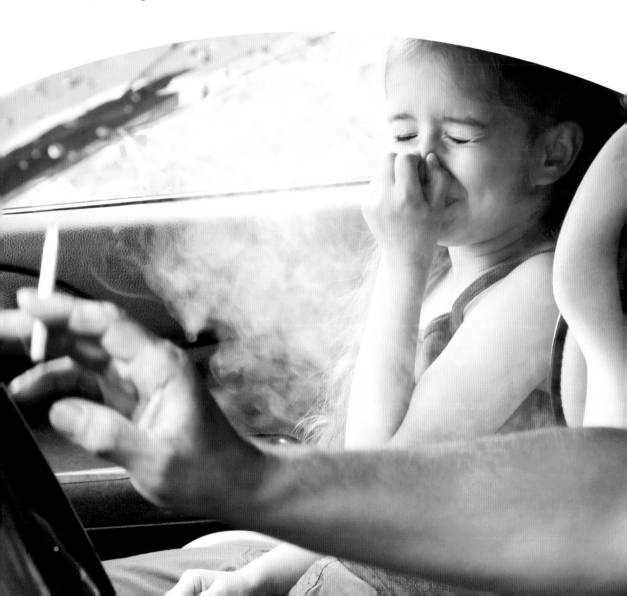

An estimated 37.8 million adults in the United States smoke cigarettes, and more than 16 million Americans are living with a smoking-related disease, costing the United States more than $300 billion annually, according to the CDC. Some researchers believe that every cigarette inhaled decreases a smoker's life expectancy by eleven minutes.

The CDC says quitting at any time can improve health, including reducing the risk for heart disease within one to two years after stopping smoking. Quitting also reduces the risk for developing certain lung diseases, including chronic obstructive pulmonary disease, which is one of the leading causes of death in the United States. Those who attempt to quit smoking often experience nicotine withdrawal symptoms such as hunger, irritability, anger, anxiety, weight gain, and clogged thinking.

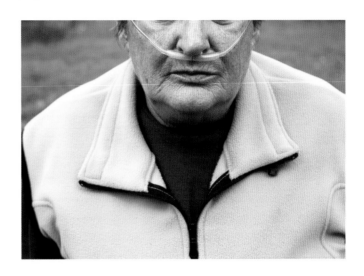

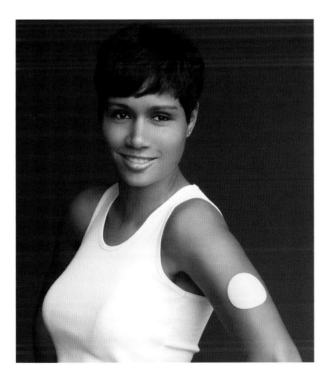

# Treatments

Those who want to quit find it helpful to seek guidance from counselors or physicians. They also try over-the-counter nicotine patches, gums, and lozenges. Physicians can also prescribe stronger nicotine patches, inhalers, and sprays, as well as some medications that don't contain nicotine. Instead, these drugs block receptors in the brain to lessen the desire to smoke. These drugs often have side effects, for example, headache, sleeping issues, gastrointestinal issues, drowsiness, and nausea.

Another treatment is hypnosis, and one study showed that hypnosis can be as effective in helping people quit smoking as nicotine patches.

# Smoking Cessation and CBD

CBD may be able to help people quit smoking, according to a study in London. The researchers found smokers using CBD reduced the number of cigarettes they consumed. This study used an inhaler, not a topical or oral administration of CBD. Participants inhaled either a placebo or CBD and were asked to inhale when they had the urge to smoke. Researchers believe CBD can alter the memories related to smoking, which can reduce the urge to have a cigarette while under stress or just craving a cigarette.

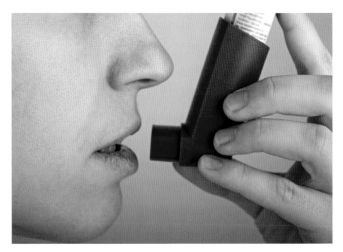

Following that study came another one in which researchers gave smokers either a dose of CBD or a placebo. Those who were given the placebo had more cravings than those with the CBD; however, the researchers were not able to show that one dose relieved withdrawal symptoms. Researchers said more studies are needed to see if using CBD for a longer period of time or at a higher dose might reduce the symptoms.

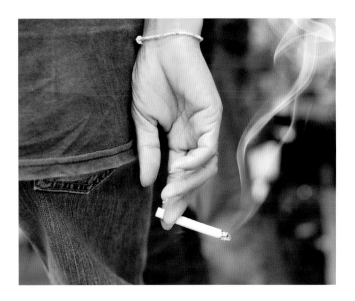

In Switzerland, people are using a cigarette made with a high concentration of CBD and a low concentration of THC instead of tobacco. The so-called CBD cigarettes are being sold in some parts of the United States as well as other countries as an alternative to smoking tobacco. In one New York City shop, customers say they are trying the CBD cigarettes as a way to quit smoking tobacco or just to find relaxation. It's a growing trend, but information on whether this practice can lead to quitting smoking tobacco is scant.

# Stroke

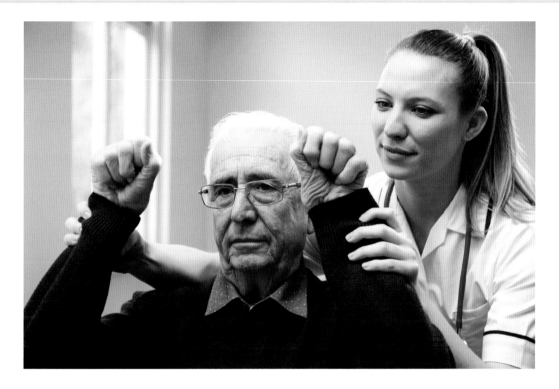

According to the American Heart Association, nearly four percent of American adults will have a stroke by the year 2030. Stroke is the fifth leading cause of death in the United States. Stroke kills roughly 140,000 Americans each year, according to the Centers for Disease Control. In addition, more than 795,000 people in the United States experience a stroke annually, with a world population experiencing about 15 million annually.

Stroke can occur to anyone at any time. It happens when the blood flow to a part of the brain gets stopped. Brain cells then get deprived of oxygen and begin to die, which can translate to loss of memory, muscle control, and other conditions. Depending on the type and severity of the stroke, people could have minor problems, lose the ability to speak, or even become paralyzed. Most people who suffer a stroke are left with some sort of disability, which could be as minor as a blind spot in the eye.

Stroke types include a hemorrhagic stroke, in which a brain aneurysm bursts or a weakened blood vessel leaks. It's the least common, and typically ends in death.

The more common stroke is called an ischemic stroke. It involves a clot that blocks blood from getting to the brain. Eighty-seven percent of strokes are ischemic. One type of ischemic stroke, called an embolic stroke, can occur with people who have atrial fibrillation, an irregular and rapid heartbeat. In this type of stroke, a clot occurs somewhere in the body and moves to the brain. Another type of ischemic stroke is a thrombotic stroke, which can occur in people who have high cholesterol and atherosclerosis, a hardening and narrowing of the arteries. Thrombotic stroke is caused by a clot that forms inside an artery that supplies blood to the brain.

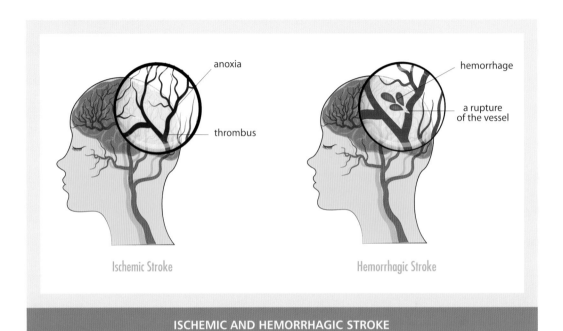

Ischemic Stroke

Hemorrhagic Stroke

**ISCHEMIC AND HEMORRHAGIC STROKE**

Another type of strike is called a transient ischemic attack that occurs when blood flowing to the brain stops. These attacks typically don't cause brain damage, but can serve as a warning that more serious strokes may occur.

Physicians diagnose stroke by considering the patient's symptoms and ordering blood and imaging tests. Symptoms while having a stroke include face drooping, arm weakness, and difficulty in speaking.

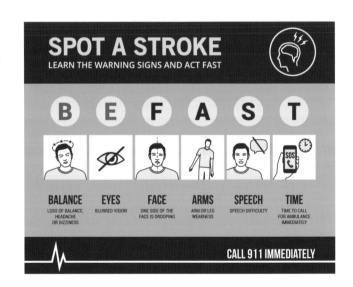

Symptoms after a stroke include weakness, pain and burning sensations; fatigue, difficulties with balance and coordination; speech problems such as being unable to understand speech, read, or write; difficult swallowing; vision problems; and depression. Recovery takes place three to four months or up to a year or two after experiencing the stroke. Some or all of these problems should improve with physical therapy and time.

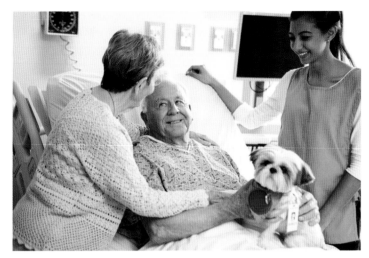

Physicians may also recommend diet change, quitting smoking, increasing exercise, and treating high blood pressure and high cholesterol. Medication also can be taken to prevent clots, and in some cases, surgery may be required. Rehabilitation is often required and could include physical therapy and working with a speech specialist; taking antidepressants and seeing a psychologist or psychiatrist.

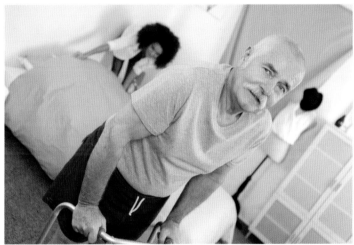

Medications often include blood thinners and anticoagulants, which can have side effects, such as bleeding that can't be stopped or easy bruising. Some of these medications also require the patient to have weekly blood tests. In addition, for the medicine to work properly, the patient will need to avoid eating certain foods with high vitamin K content, which include spinach, green tea, and kale. Some of these medications also have been linked to osteoporosis. A daily regimen of aspirin is also often prescribed.

# Prevention

Up to eighty percent of strokes can be prevented, according to the American Stroke Association.

The Harvard Medical School lists these ways to prevent stroke.

Lower blood pressure—it's the biggest contributor to stroke risk. Work toward a blood pressure of less than 135/85. Reducing salt in the diet, avoiding high-cholesterol foods, adding fruits and vegetables to your diet; getting more exercise; and quitting smoking can reduce blood pressure.

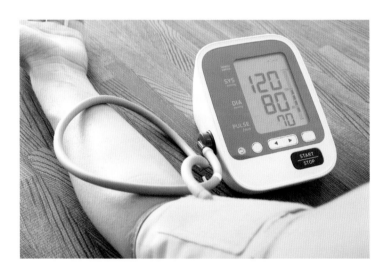

Obesity also contributes to the potential for a stroke. Even losing ten pounds could help.

Other recommendations include getting exercise at least five days weekly; drinking in moderation only; and treating diabetes and atrial fibrillation.

# Stroke and CBD

One study done on rats suggests taking CBD might help those with a certain type of ischemic stroke recover. Rats that were given CBD regained better strength and coordination compared with a control group. Another study done on rats suggested CBD might have a therapeutic effect on those with brain ischemia.

One cardiac specialist thinks CBD extracts may one day be able to be used in stroke emergency units to prevent further damage and promote healing. CBD has what are called neuroprotective effects, which can inhibit inflammation, which contributes to stroke. When someone is an emergency room with a stroke, one of the first things physician do is get the blood circulating quickly to limit brain damage. It's just a conjecture, but perhaps CBD can do the same job.

Some researchers have said they've shown that CBD can protect the brain after an ischemic stroke. But clinical studies are needed to determine the true value of CBD in treating stroke patients.

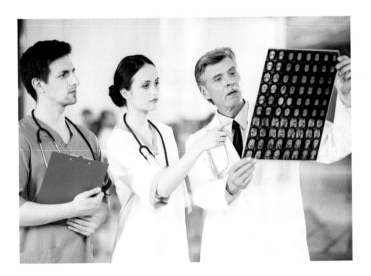

Studies also indicate that CBD might be able to help prevent stroke. CBD is said to regulate hunger; and rats were shown to have a decreased appetite when given CBD. The possibilities exist that humans can stop their desire for food by using CBD. Studies with rats also found that CBD might be able to remove plaque buildup in the arteries, which can help the body's endocannabinoid system function better. That, in turn, may slow the development of atherosclerosis, according to one researcher.

CBD has also been called a natural blood thinner—and some of the medications prescribed by physicians to thin blood can cause side effects. It's important for anyone who is at risk for stroke or has suffered a stroke to talk with a physician before adding CBD oil to the treatment plan.

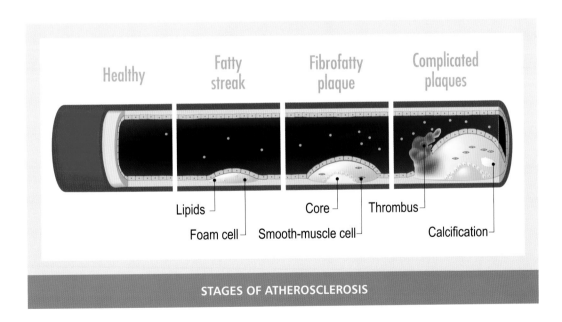

STAGES OF ATHEROSCLEROSIS

# Tinnitus

The Mayo Clinic defines tinnitus as the perception of noise or ringing in the ears. It affects about 20 percent of the United States population and is considered a symptom of a condition such as hearing loss, an injury, or a circulatory system issue.

Tinnitus can be bothersome, but typically it's not serious. It can be characterized by ringing, buzzing, roaring, clicking, or hissing in one or both ears, as well as a pulsing heartbeat like sound.

Subjective tinnitus is the kind that only you can hear and is the most common. Objective tinnitus is a rare type that a physician can hear.

Causes include problems with the nerves in your auditory pathways, damage to the inner ear cell, chronic health conditions, or injuries that affect hearing in your brain or the nerves in your ear.

Tinnitus also can be caused by hearing loss related to old age, exposure to loud noises, blockage with ear wax, and abnormal bone growth in the middle ear.

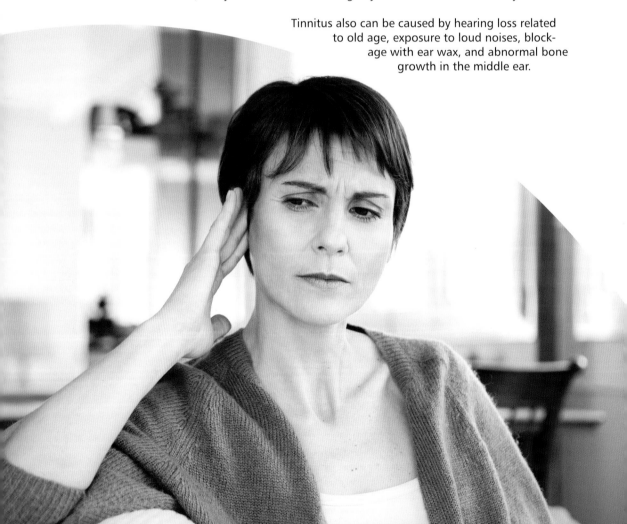